The Spirit of Nursing

The Spirit of Nursing

The Spirit of Nursing Project

Copyright © 2019 by The Spirit of Nursing Project.

ISBN:	Softcover	978-1-9845-7609-5
	eBook	978-1-9845-7608-8

All rights reserved. No part of this book may be reproduced or transmitted in any form or by any means, electronic or mechanical, including photocopying, recording, or by any information storage and retrieval system, without permission in writing from the copyright owner.

The views expressed in this work are solely those of the author and do not necessarily reflect the views of the publisher, and the publisher hereby disclaims any responsibility for them.

Any people depicted in stock imagery provided by Getty Images are models, and such images are being used for illustrative purposes only. Certain stock imagery © Getty Images.

Print information available on the last page.

Rev. date: 02/21/2019

To order additional copies of this book, contact:
Xlibris
1-888-795-4274
www.Xlibris.com
Orders@Xlibris.com
784014

Contents

Acknowledgments xv

Preface xvii

Chapter 1   When I Knew 1

Chapter 2   Nursing School Stories 25

Chapter 3   A Patient I'll Never Forget 43

Chapter 4   Collegiality & Practice 93

Chapter 5   As We Know It 123

Chapter 6   As We Remember It 133

Epilogue 143

Contributors 151

Suggested Reading 157

"When we do the best that we can, we never know what miracle is wrought in our life, or in the life of another."

Helen Keller

The Spirit of Nursing

Stories of Our Careers

Dr. Kristine Batty, Ph.D., APRN-CNP, BC-ADM, CDE, CDOE, AANP
Kelly Baxter, MS, APRN, ACHPN
Denise Bezila, MS, RN, SSGB
Patricia Bonzagni, RN
Jeannine Borozny, BS, RN, CNOR, RNFA
Dr. Rebecca Carley, DNP, APRN-CNP
Dr. Linda Del Vecchio-Gilbert, DNP, CPNP-PC, ACHPN
Dr. Robert Desrosiers, DNP, APRN, FNP-BC
Pam Dimascio, MBA, BSN, RN, CPHQ
Donna Dupuis, MS, RN
Lucille Ferrer, LPN
Leiah Gallagher, BSN, RN
Marla Goulart, MS, RN
Dr. Donna Horrocks, DNP, RN, GCNS-BC, CCRNk
Lisa Johnson, BS, RN
Rebecca L. Jones, MHA, BSN, CCM, RN
Rachel Jones, A.D.N., RN
Elaine Joyal, MSN, RN, NE-BC
Kristina Lambert, MS, APRN, FNP-BC
Linda Lambert, BS, RN
Dr. Mary Lavin, DNP, APRN-CNP
Shelley MacDonald, MS, BSN, RN
Alisha Mal, MS, RN
Michelle Mallon, MS, RN-BC
Colleen Moynihan, RN
Deborah Myers, BS, RN, CCRC
Stacie Nunziato, MSN, RN
Kathleen O'Connell, MSN, RN, CIC
Ellen O'Rourke, RN
Anabela O'Shea, BSN, RN
Dr. Darlene Noret, DNP, MSN Ed., APRN, ACAGNP-BC
Angela Quarters, BSN, RN-BC
Deborah Quirk, BS, RN
Elizabeth Raposa, MS, ACNP-BC, CCRN
Barbara Saleeba, A.D.N., RN, CRRN
Cathy Schwartz, BSN, RN, CCRN
Linda Tierney, LPN
Karen Treloar, RN, WCC
Cynthia Votto, MSN, RN
Rosemary Walker, LPN
Virginia Wilcox, MS, RN, CNML, CCRN
Dianna Wantoch, MBA, RN, CPHQ
Karen Zarlenga, BSN, RN, CDE, CDOE, CDVOE

To the patients we have cared for and
those we have yet to meet.

Acknowledgments

Editor: Allison Horrocks, Ph.D., Graduate of the University of Connecticut.

Having the dream of writing a book and turning it into one are completely different. Thank you for your expertise, time, patience and commitment in making it happen.

Illustrator: Rebekah Jean Myers, B.F.A., Graduate of Savannah College of Art and Design.

Thank you to Rebekah, who took watercolors to an idea and made it real.

Preface

When taken altogether, the contributors to this book have given more than a thousand years to the care of patients. Collectively, we have hundreds of years of disciplinary training, point of care experience, and countless sleepless nights of worry when we could not leave the job at work. We have this shared background, certainly, but we also have our own kind of shorthand: whether or not we are working at the bedside today, we still look at the veins of those around us. We do not necessarily look because we are working, or simply because it is something we have been trained to do. It is not exactly reflexive, and it's not a utilitarian look. We look at the veins because it has become an aspect of who we are, and what we share.

We look at your veins in the checkout line at the market, in the mall, in restaurants. We look at the veins because it is part of being a nurse. We confidently determine that we could "get it in" if we had the chance, and, we often talk about our successes of doing so. Most of us wouldn't turn down the chance to try. A select few among us always go for the "18," a larger gauge needle; others always preferred the "22" over any other size. Some of my colleagues confess to other habits. Turning their gaze away from the veins, they are "looking at the necks," often for possible difficulty with intubation, or thyroid disease. Some "look at hips" for difficulty with birth, or the expression on a woman's face to determine childbirth is very imminent. Others are "looking at the ankles" for signs of heart failure.

This way of looking and inhabiting the world becomes a matter of honed instinct—a funny word, really, for this habit, for it comes from the Latin instinguere, meaning in-toward and stinguere, to prick. It is something that is taught, in an empirical way, in nursing school in the course of learning about assessment. There is an objective process, and we learn how to look at the world anew, one vein, neck, and ankle at a time. But this is also, as we have discovered in sharing our stories, about a system of knowing. There is a shared world of insider knowledge nurses have, and while much of their knowledge is empirical and data driven, there is also an aspect that is less tangible and harder to name, even for those trained in precision.

Though we started collecting stories for this project in 2018, the genesis can be traced back to a graduate course that I took many years ago. I was completing a concept analysis and considering this idea that there was a shared understanding among all nurses. While struggling to explain the espirit de corps many nurses feel, I used words such as mutuality, grasping to define this professional feeling. When it came down to it, however, I asked my cohort: "We all look at people's veins, don't we?" This question elicited a strong response, with heads bobbing throughout the room. "It's part of being a nurse," they said in unison. A personal and academic interest in defining this shared sense of a spirit of nursing may have been the origin for this book, but it is a project that contains many authors and the stories of many more lives.

The contributors in this book are all nurses. Some have almost fifty years of looking and knowing, some have less than one. In recounting career highs, lows, and the mundane daily tasks that fill the months and years in between, we found that reflecting on the profession has further convinced us of this shared spirit. It is not merely the practice of nursing, but the sense of advocacy and devotion that binds us together. Many of our contributors shared how she or he knew about wanting to be a nurse. Receiving the training required to be a nurse requires commitment and choice; perhaps it is also a path that chooses you. It chooses you for your compassion, advocacy and commitment. These stories convey a love for a profession that has given back to us as much as we have given to it.

These nurses' degrees, certification and years of experience may be quantifiable. But their stories reveal that their experiences are truly incalculable. Professionally, we strive for measurable outcomes—personally, we are aware that so, so much of what we do and have done can never be measured. We have cared for persons at the beginning of life, at the end of life, and at every point in between. We also know that our difficult memories come from those we could not help. The patients who suffered, and whose families so often said: "I will never forget you." Most likely they did, but as you will see, we have not. Some of these stories about caring that we have chosen to include are difficult and heartbreaking. Others are filled with humor and reflect the buoyancy of the human spirit.

We have seen so much, felt so much, and we agree that this is what distinguishes us. In recalling these experiences, sometimes the tears returned, sometimes the laughter returned—but always, pride. In writing our stories, we hope they not only serve as validation of knowing, but as knowledge itself, so we can ask more relevant questions, think about education and perhaps approach practice differently. This collection of stories serves as a tribute to people who have had a career they are proud of. As you read their stories, you will recognize the emotion and the capacity for professionalism paired with compassion. With every encounter, we have felt it a privilege to care for someone else's loved one. As nurses, most of would honestly say we don't "drive Cadillacs in our dreams." We do, however, often wake up in a sweat, thinking we forgot to chart the 10 : 00 a.m. Lisinopril.

Much of what we experience and learn in the practice of being a nurse is not tangible, and perhaps this is why we turn to the physical triumph of inserting an I.V. as a way of marking how we enter people's lives. But there's something else that stays with us throughout our careers. An important moment in a nurse's evolution is getting her pin. Along with stories, the contributors to this book also shared their pins with one another. These items represent many of the institutions that the nurses who contributed to this volume have attended over the past half century. Some are shiny, others are deeply worn. Along with the memories and many, many stories, these pins, and the memories of our journeys, stick with us, too.

While a number of us remember using rotating tourniquets, wearing starched white caps and patients in iron lungs, the newest nurse author in this book has not even worn her pin except at graduation. The authors of this book, when asked to contribute, made it clear they didn't need credit. They also made it clear how they felt about those in their care; they were not just names on the whiteboard, or on the assignment under their name, or in an office schedule book. I, however, believe that we do, as a profession, need credit for careers and lives well lived, for caring so much about other people, and for looking at the veins.

Donna Horrocks
December 2018

Chapter One

When I Knew

*Kelly Baxter, Denise Bezila,
Jeannine Borozny, Becky Carley,
Donna Dupuis, Donna Horrocks, Lisa Johnson,
Rebecca Jones, Kristina Lambert,
Linda Lambert, Mary Lavin,
Shelley MacDonald, Michelle Mallon,
Darlene Noret, Anabela O'Shea,
Angela Quarters, Deb Quirk, Barbara Saleeba,
Diana Wantoch, Ginny Wilcox*

"The best way to find yourself is to lose yourself in the service of others."
Mahatma Ghandi

The profession of nursing was not yet one hundred years old when many of the contributors to this book first entered the field. Though people have cared for one another in times of sickness for all of human history, the idea of nursing as a career is relatively new. In the 19th century, broader cultural shifts towards institutionalized caregiving in the United States and in Europe precipitated this new field of study and form of employment as we know it today. Over time, fewer people would suffer through illness at home, and in turn, more people would live their final days in a hospital, surrounded by paid caregivers in a clinical setting. By the late 1800s, medical schools and city hospitals would eclipse older traditions of knowledge sharing and training.

As a new type of professional caregiving role became more common, nursing, as a formal career, was almost entirely composed of women. For many young women, nursing was one of a fairly small number of career paths open to them. Yet the professionals who shared their stories did not turn to nursing for lack of other options. Even if the spectrum of employment available to them was smaller than it is today, nursing was something they chose and wanted to pursue. There is a shared sense here that nursing was a field that one could be proud of, in part because it was still a part of a much longer human tradition of committing oneself to another's care.

Through personal reflections, these authors chart various pathways into their shared career. For some, the desire to become a nurse can be traced with some clarity back to a childhood event or simply a sense of knowing. These authors have just always been aware, even at a very young age, that this was how they would spend their working lives. Others were inspired by a particular interaction with a nurse, such as during a medical emergency. For some, it was the spirit of a heroic figure such as Florence Nightingale. However, not everyone can see such as a straight line from their childhood dreams to their career. For others, they can recall a desire to help others going back to a young age, yet they were less sure as to what shape that might take. Some professionals also considered similar careers, such as pharmacy, biology, microbiology, and some have even had other careers before nursing. What all of these authors share is a critical deciding moment, a point in time when the desire to be a nurse was crystallized and thought turned into action.

> *For some contributors, the path toward*
> *a career in nursing was set*
> *early—very early. Instead of seeing nursing*
> *as a career one chose,*
> *for some it is all they ever considered.*
> *Perhaps it was even destined.*

I am not sure that becoming a nurse was my destiny, but this is what my mother believed, and perhaps that is enough. I was always told that I was destined to be a nurse because of how I came into the world. My mother would explain, "the placenta was over your face when you were born," sighing as if this were the most obvious thing in the world, "it was a sign." Curiously, in following this "destiny," I would quickly learn once I had one semester in my obstetrical clinical that the placenta could not have been over my face.

Perhaps I was conceived to be a nurse. My Mom wanted to be a nurse but for many reasons was unable to do so. She highly valued the profession of nursing and believed very strongly that caring about others and helping those in need was how to make a difference in this world. She taught us as children to care for each other, work together for a cause, negotiate for what was needed, and constantly share our knowledge with each other. When it was time to make a choice for my profession, nursing clearly emphasized these strengths. Although my Mom groomed me to be become a nurse the choice was clearly mine and one I will never regret. Nursing has been such a rewarding career. I feel I have made a small difference in this world and know my life has been enriched by all the patients and colleagues who have touched my life.

Ever since I was little, I have wanted to have a career where I could help people. Nursing was always my top choice. I really did not ever think about any other occupations. I set my mind to becoming a registered nurse and after four years of nursing school, I reached that goal. It is truly as simple as that.

In retrospect, fictional companions, together with real-life friends, could play a pivotal role in childhood aspirations. From Barbie to Cherry Ames, dolls and fictional nurses could provide just enough of a stimulating interest to motivate a young person to consider nursing a career.

Growing up, I always knew. My best friend and I both loved cats and Barbie dolls. She had more of both than I could ever hope for, but we had other things in common that balanced our relationship out. We both had brothers (I had four to her one) that did not understand the attraction of the cats or the Barbie dolls. There was another aspect of our relationship that worked well: I always had to be the nurse, and she was always had to be the teacher.

In dreaming up play scenarios, it was not always easy to play nurse and teacher, but we made it work. After all, we had the cats, and they made for passable students (when they stayed still). Likewise, the Barbie dolls were great, immobile patients; Ken and Skipper were quickly added to our rosters when they came along. A turning point for me, or perhaps an escalation, was when the Barbie Registered Nurse premiered in 1961. She was simply fantastic. I was most impressed with her accessories: the navy-blue cape, white dress, hot water bottle, and diploma. Her cap didn't last long, and I never understood the heels, but then again, the metal spoon confused me, too. I still wonder what that spoon was for after more than four decades of clinical practice. At the time, the doll was marketed as representing Barbie's first career. I recall wondering why you needed more than one.

When I was young and expressed interest in nursing, my father told me it "would be a pretty good job if I ever had to get divorced." I was ten years old at the time, so I am not sure how impressed I was with that fact. I was, however, very impressed with the fictional Cherry Ames, a student nurse who was the star of more than twenty novels. Notably, Cherry Ames never got divorced. She did join the Army Nurse Corps and solved mysteries with ease. Beyond the basic outlines of her adventures, I do not recall much except perhaps the most important detail: that Cherry was a fantastic nurse. I devoured each story and to this day, remember *The Mystery in the Doctor's Office* best.

> **While fiction inspired some future nurses, a personal medical crisis would lead others toward nursing. From a painful open- heart surgery, to a prolonged treatment of a bladder tumor, to allergy shots and the polio vaccine, receiving extraordinary care at a young age would inspire some to consider a career not just as a nurse, but as a very real hero to young people in pain.**

As a child, the thought of being a nurse did not even enter my mind. I originally wanted to become an airline stewardess. But that quickly changed when I was hospitalized for open-heart surgery. As I went through this very challenging time of my life, I closely watched the team of nurses who were taking care of me. They were so kind and so very attentive to my cries of pain and frightened looks each time a procedure was to be done. That was the start of my nursing career.

From my first hospital visit at the age of five, I knew I wanted to be a nurse. It has been said that first impressions last forever, and the image of the nurse that took care of me has been deeply embedded in my memory ever since. Her starched white dress, white stockings, and white clinic shoes were complemented by a cap with a black stripe along the rim. She comforted my fears and rewarded me with vanilla ice cream and flat ginger ale, two things that I still crave when I'm not feeling well. This true "angel of mercy," and all of these small details, are lodged in my memory, forever. Who would have thought that this first encounter at the hospital would have such an influence on who I would become?

I can recall exactly when I knew I was going to be a nurse. It was not that I wanted to be a nurse; I was simply going to be one. Long after I had been toilet trained, I started to wet my pants at the age of five. My parents took me to the doctor and I was admitted to have a work-up for a bladder tumor. I will always remember how the nurses made me feel. Despite the fear, pain, and trauma of the procedures, they were always beside me. I will never forget how they indulged me—they let me have orange soda and even gave me a job at the nurses' station. As their helper, I loved pushing the prescribed button and asking, "Can I help you?" I also have less pleasant memories, and remember vividly how it took four of them to hold me down on the table. The catheterizations and fluid irrigation hurt; it was so personal, so intimate, and I always knew when they were coming. All of these aspects of my experience, the good and the bad, led me to nursing. The nurses and orange soda made for a great combination, it seems—they were heroes to me.

My story begins back when I was a child. I had many allergies when I was very young, and at the age of seven I was officially tested. I then began receiving allergy shots twice a month. I hated going to that office, so I would often hide from my mom in the hopes that the appointment would be canceled. When I inevitably made my begrudging arrival, I was always greeted with a smile by Jan, the office nurse. Jan made each visit a little less painful. Over my childhood she was always there and took an interest in my life.

I think there were several events in my young life that clearly gave me that feeling that I was born to be a nurse. I do not remember the exact date, but I do vividly remember at least three of my siblings in tow. It had to be the 1950s. I remember my mother saying over and over, "I don't care how much you cry." But that is not why I remember—that phrase was said a lot, after all. It was the other things she was saying, over and over, including her command to never, ever forget this day. I recall her other refrain: "he gave it to his own children." I remember being confused, but somehow excited.

I knew by the way the other mothers and fathers in line were crying that it was important. I knew it was not our usual Saturday morning.

Since we were headed to school on a weekend day, my older brother was convinced this was not a good situation, at least for him. My younger brothers just knew it may not be something to be happy about, selectively hearing that this was something about "medicine." If it was anything close to the Castor Oil it was going to be painful. All in all, we stood in line a long time. I found a lot of this morning to be strange, yet exciting. On this day, the children who were upset by the prospect of getting medicine were not comforted by their parents. I now realize that no amount of screaming was getting us back in the station wagon without the polio vaccine.

In the days before that Saturday, my mother would get teary when she talked about the possibility of no more children needing the March of Dimes. I never understood why a dime would help people walk. In my childhood, a fear of polio, the word "crippled," and the lingering threat of the "summer virus" were always being discussed. Still, when I was vaccinated, I was too young to understand the implications of what was happening. But I know my parents instilled in me, just by their actions that day, that there was a man who believed in the truth he had found, enough to give this discovery to his own children. That was enough for my mother and all of the other mothers in lines, all over the world.

This experience inspired a desire to know more. I couldn't put this longing into words at the time. I now know that it was a craving to understand what the disease did to people who contracted it, and how they needed special care after having the virus. I also couldn't call it "wanting to be a nurse" at the time, but I know it was. There would be many other times as a child I would have this feeling of wanting to know much more than what I was being told. It was always about sickness, disease, and how people felt when they were sick and why. A simple virus in the family would set me into motion of asking so many questions I needed to be stifled. I do, however, give credit to my parents for the important aspects of that Saturday. Without ever meeting him, or knowing anything more than what they had learned from having children about disease management, my parents knew they had the opportunity to save their children from a devastating virus. There would be many more days growing up when I knew how my mother and father felt about important things. This was just one of them.

Watching how a nurse cared for a friend, family member, or neighbor had a profound impact on other future nurses. Whether it was the demonstration of empathy or a burning desire to understand a complex medical situation, these writers understood at a young age that a profession of caring was for them based on the examples of others.

During the summer between my seventh and eighth grade years, I broke my ankle. Since I was in a cast all summer, I was limited with what activities I could do and spent a lot of time indoors. During that same summer, my grandfather was diagnosed with throat and neck cancer. He had a radical neck surgery to remove the cancer. While he stayed with my family in our home to recuperate, I became very impressed with the visiting nurse. She was caring, empathetic, and compassionate, not just to my grandfather but the entire family. The nurses who cared for my ankle and for my grandfather helped me to decide that I was going to be a nurse. I always knew I wanted to be part of a profession that gives back to the community, and nursing was that perfect fit.

My mom was a nurse and a role model for compassionate, person-centered care. When I was young, she worked in a segregated southern community. This was the 1960s. One of the families she worked with was African American; they were tenant farmers. I don't know how they met, but I remember going with her to their house on a nearby tobacco farm. My mom helped them when she could. We would leave items they needed at the door; she never wanted to make a spectacle of it. She always touched her friend and the children, calling them by name and asking something personal. It was her way of showing she cared.

We would frequently get invited over to eat with them and we usually did. In the 1960s, politically and socially, this was unusual, but it was genuine for this family and mine. I always wanted to be a nurse, but not just any nurse— one like my mom. The memories of going with her and observing her servant's heart impacted me in so many ways.

When I was very small, my father was deployed and we went to stay with my paternal grandmother in Florida. My mother went to work as a nurse on a maternity unit in the city hospital. There were many patients who received welfare assistance; often, the patients did not have insurance. Years later, a colleague of my mother's (who was an OB-GYN fellow at the time) told me a story about Mom.

In the late 1950s, it was the hospital's practice not to give medication to the delivering women who received welfare. Learning of this, my mother was incensed. She was ex-military and used to equal treatment of delivering mothers. On her own, my mother started paying for the medication these women needed. The administration told her to stop and she told them they would have to fire her. The doctors and other nurses where so ashamed that they had done nothing that they helped get the policy changed.

This colleague of my mother's told me that she taught him more about caring for people than all his years in medicine. I wasn't surprised by this story, since I had witnessed her advocacy firsthand as a child. This memory helped solidify what a nurse should be in my mind. It also started me on a path of working with people who are homeless, which has continued for over 30 years.

This story is not mine, but it is one I have recorded and received permission to share. A colleague recently told me about the exact moment she knew she "had to be a nurse." She was a young wife. Her husband complained of a headache. To relieve some pain, he took a shower. It was in that shower that he died of a cerebral hemorrhage. He was 21 years old. She describes the events as passionately as I have heard her before, but this time it was not a stranger's story. With deep emotion in her eyes, she describes these painful moments, not for the sake of telling, but to explain something about herself. With gratitude, she describes what he left her, a son. But along with those details, comes something perhaps serendipitous: the "calling." After what happened to him, she knew that moment she had to be a nurse. This person is impressive in so many ways—as a nurse, a colleague, and a friend. But perhaps what is most awesome about her is how she emerged and grew from tragedy. She became a caregiver because of her loss and after beginning again, raised a wonderful daughter to become one, too.

I knew I wanted to be a nurse when I was about seven years old. At the time, I was fascinated with medical issues, but I obviously had no real understanding of them. I know how to plot this story with some precision because this is the time when I met Mrs. B. This woman living in my aunt's neighborhood conjured a strange combination of fascination and respect within me.

Looking back, I think she had Polio, but it was never described as that. I met her on one of our many trips we took on Sundays to visit my mother's only sister, my aunt Bet. This twenty-minute ride seemed much longer because it was difficult to get all of us children to settle down and ride without fighting. These otherwise boring biweekly trips soon became my chance to beg my cousin to take me to her friend Amy's house. Amy was nice enough, but she was hardly the main attraction. This was about getting to see Amy's mother, the apparently first-nameless-Mrs. B. and the Iron Lung she was encased in.

This Iron Lung—this magnificent thing—was right in the middle of the B. family living room. Amy was one of three children that could usually be found in this same room, busy planets orbiting their sun. Mrs. B. could talk from within the Iron Lung, but only when she exhaled. Walking into the home, we could usually hear something along the lines of, "Bobby, Jimmy, Amy, pick up your rooms!" followed by an audible breath in. Then, "Joe, I'll need a drink soon," and another breath. One of the greatest surprises for me was that Amy and the others usually did what she said, and immediately.

I was not the only one who was surprised by this. My own mother seemed to use this whenever she couldn't get control of us, noting, "Mrs. B.'s kids follow directions right from an Iron Lung, and I can't get you kids to do anything." My siblings were unsurprisingly nonplussed by this comparison. They were also far less interested in Mrs. B. beyond the fact that she was seemingly trapped inside a medical device. "Really," they'd ask, exasperated, "she NEVER comes out of that?" Or, the ever-popular question, "how does she, you know, go?" For them, it was "gross." I didn't think it was gross; I was completely taken by the whole concept of someone living in this tube. I was also admittedly a bit annoying in my own way. I wanted to know everything about her—the why, how, and when—even when the other kids grew tired of talking about it. I was plainly told, "she had a virus that left her this way, that's all." I recall thinking that I once had a virus and threw up for two days, yet I was not living in a tube with only a mirror to look at. We visited my family and by extension, the B. family, as often as my parents could take the ride in the station wagon with the wood on the sides. It was never often enough for me.

One day we got a call from aunt Bet. Mrs. B. had gotten sick; she'd had a high fever, gone to the hospital, and died. I had so many more questions, all of which went unanswered. In the end, though, Mrs. B. made a more lasting impact on me than she could have ever imagined. As a mother, I can't image living my life with a voice that could only be heard when the machine allowed, or just seeing my reflection from that tube. I do know one important thing I realized (and I know my mother did, too) : the love Mrs. B. had for her children, and the respect they had for her. I thank her for sparking an interest that still has not died out in me.

> *Role models come in many forms for nurses—some are relatives who live close to us and others are historical figures from long ago. From a beloved mother and aunt to Clara Barton and Florence Nightingale, the paths tread by extraordinary and ordinary nurses have inspired many careers.*

At first blush there are maybe fifty adjectives that come to mind. Realistically, though, when I think of my rewarding vocation, the top words that I focus on are the inner self, compassion, empathy, and the caregiver. At times, a nurse provides comfort, a simple touch, or a smile in your eyes. All of these are part of reaching out to another human being to make life more serene, transcending above and beyond the technology.

More than thirty years ago, I began college studies for my nursing career. I was a wife, mother, daughter, and grand-daughter. I was pursuing the career I always had intentions of following after high school, but that had been out of reach financially to that point. My career afforded me the availability to explore different types of caregiving, from a novice on a step-down cardiac unit to maternal child care, community nursing, emergency care, oncology, and hospice. All of these jobs were very diverse, pushing me to draw upon knowledge I had acquired to provide the best quality of care, sometimes with a little assertion necessary in order to advocate for your client when necessary.

It was not until much later, perhaps more than a dozen years into my career, that I realized the impact of my example of caregiving. In her senior year of high school, my daughter announced that she intended to pursue a nursing career. She also worked more than a dozen years prior to advancing her career. Upon her recent graduation from her Nurse Practitioner program she wrote to me:

> You have really and truly made it possible for me to get where I am and be who I am today. Like so many of my Nurse Practitioner classmates, from a young age we watched our moms demonstrate what it means to be a nurse. For me it was stopping by a patient's home for an 'emergency home care' visit, while we were out and about because there was a need.
>
> I remember you caring for this patient when the HIV/AIDS crisis was barely spoke of. You nursed him with compassion and without judgement. I recall you driving an hour and a half when he was in crisis and in need of IV therapy. I know that he and his mom were so grateful for your presence. I read numerous cards of thanks and was too young to really realize the comfort you provided.
>
> The pediatric patient that felt comfort in knowing the nurse changing his central line dressing was not going to experience a painful day, if a nurse he did not know arrived, but rather a gained bond of trust. This patient was not much younger than I, possibly 6 -7 years, but I remember how delighted they were to see you and meet me when we were invited to a Birthday party. I can't imagine how difficult it was as both a mother and a nurse to care for terminally ill children, but I know you did it

well by the way all of those families reacted when you extended yourself to them, so their child would have comfort with their home care nurse.

Whenever I talk about my mother as a nurse, I really think about the example you set—the caring, the proficiency and the ability to let your patients into your heart. I also think about how you did all of this as a single mom.

I am really proud to say watching you care for your patients and their families has inspired me and guided me in my own practice.

As I share pieces of this beautiful note, I know that supporting her to fulfill her dream was important. I have had the privilege of caring for many beautiful children, adults, as well as providing support to their extended family.

The moment I knew I wanted to be a nurse occurred when I was about eight years old. I was visiting my nana, who had eight children—seven sons and one daughter. My aunt, the lone daughter, was going to nursing school at the time. Occasionally, she would leave her nursing uniform in her bedroom. I would sneak into her room, where she also kept her stethoscope and nursing cap, and I would not-so-secretly put them on. After carefully pinning my hair up, I would look in the mirror at my reflection. Inspired by the show Emergency! I would pretend I was nurse "McCall." I usually got caught. My nana would yell to me, telling me to take my aunt's nursing cap off and put her stethoscope back. No matter how many times I was told, I would try and sneak back to don the cap and stethoscope.

My early interest in nursing came partially from this kind of play and fantasy. But it was also based on a desire to make people feel the way I did when my mother nursed me. She would put a cool cloth on my head when I had a fever. Her caring touch was better healing than any other medication. As I matured, so did my interest in nursing. At sixteen, I was introduced to the role of the certified nursing assistant. I started a clinical training at an emergency department, and I became responsible for assisting a male nurse. I made suture kits, stocked the equipment in the department, and took patients to the x-ray machine. I thought I was the best. With this job, I was able to watch and listen to the medical and nursing staff. Impressed with what a difference they made, I was excited to be in that environment. It brought me back to that feeling of care and love from my mom when I was ill.

That's when I really knew my destiny. From that point forward, I was determined to help people in need, whether that meant dealing with a serious problem or offering a smile and some conversation. It did not hurt that I finally got to wear the uniform, either.

If you were to ask me why I became a nurse, I would have to say that I wanted to be a part of a profession that was highly respected and looked up to by many. As a young girl I read books on Clara Barton and Florence Nightingale. I was inspired by their focus on caring for individuals who were incapacitated, either by injury and illness, as well as their displays of compassion and strength. Both women were nurses as well as strong leaders, educators, scientist and researchers.

Florence Nightingale was a trailblazing figure in nursing. She became a pioneer of policy. I feel a strong connection to her, like so many of my colleagues. She was known for her night rounds to aid the wounded, establishing her image as the 'Lady with the Lamp.' During the Crimean War, she and a team of nurses improved the unsanitary conditions, reducing mortality. Nightingale made it her mission to improve practices, at times lowering the death rate by two-thirds. She tirelessly devoted her life to ensuring safe, but compassionate care for those deserving. To this day, she is broadly acknowledged and revered in nursing.

I am proud to say that I have been a nurse for the past forty years and have had the privilege of providing care to many patients and their families. I will always advocate for the profession of nursing to anyone who is considering it. As a nurse I still continue the work started by both Clara Barton and Florence Nightingale. I have opportunities to be a caregiver, patient advocate, leader, educator, author, scientists and / or researcher, just to name a few. I am a member of a highly regarded profession. Despite there being so many more choices of career, I am truly proud to be a nurse and would do it all over again.

Though more and more men are entering nursing, it has been, and still is a female-dominated profession. Historically, many women felt that this was one of a small number of paths open to them. Yet even the women who felt that their options were relatively limited still saw nursing as a path one chose, not one that was chosen for them.

As a young girl, my mother told me that I could do and be anything I wanted. I was the youngest of two, arriving after my brother. After I finished high school, I went away to begin my university studies. Once there, I was surrounded by (mostly) brainy boys who all were acing Chemistry classes and the other sciences needed for the pre-medicine track. I had been a straight-A student all my life, but something about being away from home, surrounded by science and math "geeks" made me wonder if this was really for me.

In the middle of my sophomore year, I took a semester off to think things over. I used that time to apply to nursing schools around the country, including where I grew up. While working as a waitress and camp counselor, I learned that I got into several schools, including one that geographically could not have been farther away from me. The following autumn, I enrolled in the nursing program. I rented a small (supposedly) winterized cottage and became a serious student once again. I knew I wanted to help other people, and that nursing would give me a pathway to do that. I attended all my classes, completing and even enjoying the mandatory sciences. With this curriculum, organic chemistry and physics were interesting because they explained how things happened—the same with anatomy, physiology, psychology, and child development. There was so much to know about how our bodies and mind worked and who we become who we are.

As I completed each nursing rotation, I was excited and nervous at the same time. Halfway through one of my medical-surgical rotations, my instructor told us: "You never guess an answer or make it up. If you don't know something, you say, 'I don't know, but I will find out.'" That has stuck with me. It made sense—we were dealing with people's lives, after all. We had a big responsibility and it should not be taken lightly. I still try to remember that wisdom when I don't know the answer to something.

I continued to learn through my clinical rotations. Clinical rotations helped me make the best decision: quit smoking cigarettes. I wondered how I could take care of others and teach them how to stay well yet I was not following the same advice. In the end, I graduated with honors and was asked to give a speech at the commencement ceremony. I felt honored and spoke of our role to help and treat others as you would want your own family members to be treated. I also stressed the point that I learned we should never forget to care for ourselves as well.

As I look back on my career of more than three decades, I realize that so much of my nursing training prepared me for the challenges that lay ahead in life. As the nurse in the family, I cared for my mother, brother, and father, who came to the end of their lives in that order. They faced serious illnesses, some longer than others, and they shared their end of life wishes with me along the way. I helped my family to achieve most of them; some were easier than others, but I tried my best and they did, too. I will be forever grateful for the time I had with them—for the good times and the toughest times. Being a nurse has helped me sincerely appreciate every day that my family and I have been able to do what we set out to do. Life is short, but caring for yourself and others enhances it in so many ways. That means a lot from a girl who was told she could be and do anything.

When I was young, I was totally convinced I would become a French teacher, despite my mom being a nurse. My father had other ideas, and insisted I become a nurse for the U.S. Navy. I never became a French teacher, nor did I join the Navy, but I did become a nurse. My mom was so proud. She talked a lot about her own sister being a nurse, describing how their father had to fix up the attic for her to study. I was in the sixth grade when it happened. I realized that nursing would take a lot of studying, but it would be worth it. I saw the pride my mom had for her sister, who is now 94 years old.

In my journey of becoming a nurse, I moved along a path from candy striper (volunteer) to registered nurse (RN). Over several decades, I have worked in Oncology, Emergency Nursing, and Intensive Care units in a community hospital. One difficulty working in a community hospital is caring for patients you know as neighbors. I have realized that you do not care more or less when your patient is someone you know. The Johnny is a great equalizer in that way. I have loved what I have done for the past 37 years. While I do not have any regrets about abandoning the dream of teaching French, I do wish I had pursued a career as a Navy nurse.

I remember my decision to become a nurse happened while I was in high school. In my day, women were teachers or nurses. I had no idea of the impact of this decision on my life, or the openness and honesty that people would afford me in my career. Deciding to become a nurse is something I did a long time ago. Yet I realize new dimensions of just how right this decision was for me over and over again in my practice.

As a new nurse, there were so many incidents that brought new insight and awareness of people's needs. I remember the sadness while caring for my first patient with terminal cancer. He had a wife and two small children. I know my support of him and his wife helped them all to get through this difficult time. In those early years, I cared for many patients with quadriplegia, cancer, vascular disease, and diabetes. These and other patients suffered complications that are no longer even seen due to amazing changes in health care management.

Little did I know just how all-encompassing the role of the nurse could be, even off the clock. Everywhere I went, I might have someone ask me the meaning of a diagnostic test, what high LDL means, what foods had the most iron, and so on. Of course, all of this was before Google and Siri entered our lives. But seriously, I felt that offering people an understanding of medicine was an important aspect of my role. Thus began my "career" as neighborhood nurse. Over the years, I have had so many experiences with friends and their families. I recall running down the street before the ambulance would arrive to intervene with a neighbor who had fallen, driving a family member to the emergency room after a rescue wagon left, looking at wounds and rashes, and running to the hurt child on a baseball field. Friends who had dying family members would call and ask me what to expect. They would want to know if I could come and see how close someone was to "the end," when what they really needed was another person to be with them, to help guide them, to assure them that they were not alone. I have listened to stories of anxiety and depression; I've shared in others' feelings of powerlessness and their elation over good news.

Looking back at my life, I am so lucky to have chosen nursing as my profession. Growing up there was not as many career choices as there are today. Many of my friends wanted to be teachers or secretaries. Only a handful expressed an interest in nursing. As for me, I really did not know where I could make a difference. In fact, when I really began to lean toward a nursing career, my guidance counselor discouraged me because I was "not very strong in the sciences."

But I had gotten a taste of the hospital setting by working as a candy striper (volunteer) and as I sat with patients and helped to comfort them, I knew what I wanted. I applied to nursing school despite the objection of my guidance counselor. I was accepted, and have never regretted that decision.

To me, nursing is totally about making the connection with your patient. The patient must feel confident in you, know you care about them, and trust you. Without that connection there can be a tendency to drift away from what is most important, the patient. As I reflect upon my nursing career, I remember many special patients.

There was the 11-year-old who was struck by a car while riding his bike. He was paralyzed from the neck down, had a tracheostomy, and was admitted to our Intensive Care Unit many times. During one admission he became anxious and conveyed that something was wrong. Although the doctor was at the bedside, this young boy asked for me, mouthing that I would "know what to do." That moment was unforgettable. I knew at that point it wasn't all about being strong in the sciences.

Go into nursing? At age 18 the answer was "No." The next phase of my life was marriage, children, and life experiences. At age 30, the answer was "Not really sure." I actually wanted to be a travel agent, but that seemed unlikely as my family was growing. I did eventually start my journey to become a nurse. Next came schooling, a new baby boy to our family, and the stress of figuring out how to get this all done. Our family survives the next five years as I graduate college, my oldest daughter graduates high school, and my little boy starts kindergarten.

I begin my nursing career at a small community hospital I loved from the very beginning. Orientation as a new nurse was interrupted as my father collapses with an MI 600 miles away. I make a promise to my Dad, in the ICU, that I will make him so proud and I will be the best nurse I can be. I did just that, with help along the way, and great mentors encouraging me. I found my love in Rehabilitation Nursing and never looked back, not even to being a travel agent. I learned that I really did want to be a nurse, to make a difference for my patients and staff I work with. I recently ended my career as a rehabilitation nurse, but I finished with the best team possible. I know what it means to have all the wonderful memories of a job well done. Hope you are proud Dad.

Family members and colleagues can inspire one another—often more than they know. Even after completing a degree or other accomplishment in nursing, sometimes seeing a peer excel is what makes a career feel right.

Growing up, I had a friend named Ellen. Our fathers worked together at a telephone company and they wanted both of us to be nurses. My own father did not approve of me "seeing men's bodies," a fact he made abundantly clear. I had to keep reminding him it didn't matter what part of the body I could see, I wasn't really looking. At any rate, both Ellen and I went on to nursing school. We both graduated and went into different specialties, but we carried the same pride of our nursing school days. Nearly forty years later, as we write this story, we admit to still feeling emotional about that time.

While I pursued a career in Oncology, Ellen went into pediatrics. I always knew my friend would thrive as a pediatric nurse. On one particular day, she not only showed me her skill with children, but her commitment to a colleague. It's not a miracle story, or a saving a life story, but to me, it felt like it was.

I had only been home from the hospital for a week with my baby girl but we were both crying uncontrollably. Any nurse or mother will tell you that colic is not pleasant for the new mother or the infant. I was crying along with my daughter from exhaustion. Then Ellen appeared, with bottles of Orange Crush in tow for me. She poured the Orange Crush, took that baby in her arms, and showed me her skill. Some might say she was able to get the baby to sleep because she wasn't the one who was exhausted or hormonal. I don't think so. She truly had found her gift in pediatrics. I know that as much as I know I found my gift in her.

Nursing has been so much more than a profession for me; it is a way of life. What a tremendous opportunity to connect with individuals in such a real way in times of vulnerability, fear, uncertainty or joy. Most people want to be heard, validated, and genuinely cared for. In my years of practice in palliative and hospice care, I have had the great fortune to meet people who are at very fragile moments in life. I have found in these moments that they are often reflective, thoughtful, and prioritize things in a much different manner. I have learned so much from these encounters with "strangers," experiences that I will never forget. It is an honor to care for the sick and dying. It is the human connection of care and surpasses all boundaries. It is an opportunity to provide compassion and dignity to another human being. What a privilege!

I come from a family of nurses with my mother, aunts, and cousins choosing this noble profession for their life work. Although we have all worked in different settings with different patient populations, we are connected through our experiences of caring for the sick. The joyful and sorrowful patient stories that we share allow us to bond on a deeper level. I cannot imagine another profession that would fill my soul like nursing does. As I prepare for the completion of my doctoral work in nursing, I look forward to the decades of nursing work ahead of me and am excited about the continued opportunity to learn and grow in this wonderful profession.

Taking on a career in nursing can also be a shrewd, practical choice, especially for women seeking to balance a career with family. Sometimes, nursing is a career that emerges along the way to something else entirely.

I was born in the Azores and I came to the United States at an early age. Education was never a priority in my family. I was the first to graduate high school and the first to go to college. In all that time, I never had any plans of becoming a nurse. When I was enrolled as a student at a university, I wanted to be a high school history teacher. I had a part-time job as a secretary at a nursing home while I was working on my degree, and this was the first time I considered nursing. Since I was a staff member, I had the chance to go to nursing school and get reimbursed for tuition, books, and fees.

All I had to do was maintain a C average. I decided to give nursing a try; if I liked it that would be great. If I did not, my degree had been free. In 2005, I became an LPN. Two years later, I became an RN, and in 2018 I received my BSN. Since 2005, I have worked in a nursing home as well as in an emergency department, the surgical arena and most recently, in an intensive care unit. I have met patients who have touched my life, but sometimes more importantly, changed the way I view certain things. I have also met patients and colleagues who have made me second guess my career. I have seen many things and worked with some people who hate their jobs. I have told myself that if I ever got to that point, I would find something else to do.

That has been the beauty of nursing: there are so many specialties to try. Typically, it is the ones you are most scared to jump into that end up being the most gratifying. In these thirteen years, I have worked alongside novice and highly experienced nurses, and each one of them has played a role in making me the nurse I am today. Nursing afforded me the ability to raise my children while working various shifts to accommodate family needs. I am grateful for all of the encounters I've had. Nursing may not have been part of my original plan, but becoming a nurse has been one of my greatest achievements.

Nursing was not my first thought as a career. I originally wanted to work in Special Education. After an aunt suggested the nursing career, I changed my mind quickly.

In my first job as a nurse, I distinctly remember my head nurse. She had the white uniforms, stockings, and nurses cap; she was tough but fair. She was on the unit always-helping staff and ensuring patients had everything thing they needed. I learned what being a leader meant from her.

I think that life, in general, is the same as nursing. They both need teamwork and the collaboration of different people with different titles working for the same goal. I have been very fortunate to work throughout my hospital career to be side by side with groups of people who work for the same goal. What is important is that we work in harmony with one another and for a purpose.

Chapter Two

Nursing School Stories

Jeannine Borozny, Leiah Gallagher,
Marla Goulart, Donna Horrocks,
Rebecca Jones, Colleen Moynihan, Karen Treloar

"Your vision of where or what you want to be is the greatest asset you have. Without having a goal it's difficult to score."

Paul Arden

What does it take to become a nurse? Some of the nurses featured in this book always knew that this was the right profession for them. Others saw an opportunity at just the right time or experienced a trauma that led them to want to care for people. After making that critical decision to become a nurse, all of these writers discovered that there is so much more to do and to learn. No matter their path into the profession, all of the nurses who shared their stories for this collection received more than one kind of education. All had to learn at the point of care and in a classroom.

Looking back at their earliest training, some remember caring for an ill parent or an opportunity in high school. Nurses of an earlier generation also recall starting clinical rotations rather early in life, with some taking on challenging cases in clinical when they were still teenagers. Today, a two to four-year degree program that includes a series of clinical rotations is often the standard, but that historically has not always been the case. Much has changed, particularly of the past few decades, with regards to nursing education. No matter when the contributing nurse started her clinical, however, each recalls the initial fear, trepidation, and excitement at having the chance to finally practice.

Nurses are no longer expected to wear starch white uniforms, colorful capes, or carefully positioned caps. The shoe requirements are not quite as strict as they once were, but the standards remain high otherwise. There are also physical things they no longer carry with them that are detailed in this book. Generally, nursing students today are not the aspiring "women in white." Yet many of these professionals share common experiences: the stress of learning the necessary sciences, the pressure to perform well on standardized testing and credentialing exams, and so forth. There is also a shared emphasis on finding good mentors and learning from patients.

As these stories suggest, nursing school is more than a place or institution one attends. In this chapter, it is clear that one does not become a nurse simply by passing enough time in a classroom, library, or clinical ward. There is not a single examination run by a school or accreditation board that can truly make a nurse (though getting a degree and passing the right exams is also necessary). Nursing school, in the end, is a process. It is about the feeling of becoming a professional who has the technical skill and that something more—that spirit of caring—that is harder to quantify.

Some of the authors in this collection attended nursing school more than fifty years ago. Others graduated just this past year. Whether their training began at home, in high school, or at a four-year institution, all nursing students quickly understand just how much there is to be learned.

When asked how many years I have been a nurse, I am never sure how to reply. I say 47 but I know it's much more than that. As a young child I remember frequently taking care of a close relative who was sickly. I remember getting her aspirin, making her a very hot cup of tea, and offering her a bandana to "squeeze out" an intense headache. I would run to the bathroom as she frequently wretched over the toilet.

When I went to nursing school and learned about alcoholism, I realized she probably did not have migraines. We never used that term in my family. It was nursing school that taught me the terminology, and how to pick up the pieces of a cracked and broken home. I know now that many nurses are children of alcoholic parents. I wonder how many didn't realize it until nursing school. I was one of seven children, many nieces, and nephews—I remember caring for all of them, the diapers, feeding, and much more. I think I have been a caregiver all of my life.

At the age of sixteen, I had the opportunity to enter a nurses' aide program at a local chronic disease hospital. Today, it would be called a skilled nursing facility. After that, when I graduated high school, I applied to LPN school. This was a dream come true. By this time, I had already witnessed the outcomes of severe disease, poorly diagnosed cancers, spinal cord injuries, Parkinson's disease, many birth defects, and Multiple Sclerosis. I have a particularly vivid memory of two young men, both in their thirties, who had terminal metastatic brain cancer and were in the hospital at the same time, together. What I remember most is the faces of their wives. They had sad, fake smiles; I call them the grief smiles. The pain of these smiles stayed with me. I was too young and immature to know how to react because I was too young to know how to handle it for myself. Now I know I could only be the shoulder for them to cry on. Back then, I didn't have a shoulder big enough to handle it.

Other patients were challenging as well. I remember my charge nurse trying to make sure I couldn't see some of the procedures. With one in particular, I wanted nothing more than to see behind those curtains. I wanted to see the man who was losing his face to cancer. I was shielded from some of this, but not other traumas. I was at work the night my next-door neighbor hemorrhaged to death. Technically, it was lung cancer. I remember him desperately reaching for containers to cough the blood into. Often this meant a wastebasket, urinal, or cup. Most of all, I remember his ashtray, filled with clotted blood. The clots held his extinguished cigarettes together and still, he was smoking. At that time, almost everyone smoked. This was the first patient I had to do post-mortem care on. Most of us who have been nurses for more than 40 years can relate to this. Those who have not must wonder why we didn't know, why we couldn't stop ourselves or others.

Being the oldest child in my family, I have always tended to be the responsible type. I developed a caregiver mentality early on. Then, as I grew older and entered high school, I was very much influenced by the Sisters of Mercy who taught me. They encouraged an attitude of doing for others. Under their instruction, I learned that whatever career choice I made, I was not just selecting a job but a vocation, a calling. While I was exploring what my future might hold, I was made aware that a local hospital was recruiting high school volunteers. They would call the group "The Marion Club." Many young girls joined the group and were trained by an RN in the basics of nursing care. After a year of training, at the age of 16 we were hired for the summer. This marked the beginning of my nursing career.

I started nursing school in September of 1967. I found the world of nursing to be so different than I had imagined. We were taught from the first minute: the patient is number one, and we were to care for them and about them as if they were family. I spent countless hours studying, doing care plans, and taking on multiple rotations of shifts at nursing venues. Living in a dormitory was also a learning experience. We all had to learn how to live with different personalities. Three years later, I graduated. My colleagues and I were able to place that one-inch black velvet on our caps. This was the sign I had been waiting for. I had finally made it.

Throughout my time in nursing school, it was weirdly comforting to know that every student in my class was going through the exact same thing. We were all stressed out of our minds non-stop. It did not matter who it was, we could all vent to each other and be reassured that we all had the same worries.

I was 22 years old and sitting in my first nursing class when a professor asked me to introduce myself in a way that would be effective for patient care delivery. I gave my name and explained that I was not born in the United States, and further, that English was my third language. After all the student introductions, the professor explained that those who were not native to countries with English as the primary language would never be effective communicators.

By extension, such nurses would be unable to deliver safe, high quality care to patients. She also went on to say that ineffective communication was a major reason for medical errors; this problem could be attributed, she said, to individuals delivering care who did not primarily speak English. The professor then turned to me and asked, "are you understanding what I am saying?" I was speechless and I felt as small as a bug. I was very afraid I would cause patient harm because I was not born in the United States.

I went to speak to the professor after class. I was immediately dismissed and told that if I wanted to speak to her, I would have to sign up for an appointment during office hours. This situation went on for about two weeks. After that I attempted to speak with the Dean of Nursing, who thought the situation was very funny. I was told to not be so "sensitive" and that if I did some research, I would find than medical errors are strongly related to ineffective communication. I felt demeaned once again. At that point, I was about to quit nursing altogether.

Then I met with a friend who had graduated from high school with me and I explained how disheartened I was with this nursing program. I felt that nursing was not for me because I did not want to hurt anyone. This friend encouraged me to meet with the instructors of a local diploma program. This was the best advice I have ever followed. I have now been a nurse for over a decade. I have effectively cared for my patients and advocated for their needs. I truly love being a nurse and it is the most professionally fulfilling career I could ever imagine having.

> *Most nurses today can be found in colorful scrubs, their heads bare, and wearing whatever shoes make the most sense for their feet. Those who attended nursing school years ago, however, have distinct memories of strict uniform standards and of course, the icing on the cake: the nursing cap.*

When I think of nursing school, I think of my nurse's cap. We were told it would "keep your hair neatly in place." In reality, it looked a lot like something a maid would wear. The caps with wings made it appear as though novice nurses might take flight at any moment. Aesthetics aside, far from keeping anything in place, the cap was often falling off of your head, or falling into other things. Some of those things they fell into we didn't want to think about. Thankfully, the cap that resembled a cupcake could be washed, you just had to dry it with a towel stuffed inside.

The nurses' cap really meant something to those of us who had one. I will never forget putting the black ribbon on the "cupcake" just before graduation. We stood taller and walked prouder; I honestly thought the cap made us professionals.

It is easy to laugh about the nurses' cap today, but many of us were extremely proud to wear it. All through nursing school, we waited for the ultimate goal: getting that black stripe. The nurse's cap represented the hard work I had done to enter the profession. I know patients admired it; I know families acknowledged it, they recognized us as who we were. And despite its impracticality, I was so very proud to wear it. I have heard some nurses describe wearing the cap as a horrible thing; they are all happy the cap-wearing days are gone. That could not be further from the truth for me. I know some colleagues who still wear theirs on nurses' day. Those of us who had to wear them for many years still smile at the sight. The smile is very similar to why we look at the veins.

I understand why the cap was phased out and then eliminated altogether in the early 1980s. One very obvious reason was that these caps were hard to keep white. Many people smoked on the job; there were times when you followed the doctor down the hallway of the ward with an ashtray. Visitors could also smoke in the patients' rooms. Most of our caps became yellow from smoking at the nurses' station. For this reason alone, perhaps it was wise to eliminate them.

My nursing school uniform was not attractive. I liked the other schools' uniforms more than my own. A starched white pinafore with green stripes was just not a good look. But there were other problems. Fashion aside, the students in my program could be spotted from a mile away between the white pinafore and the cupcake on our heads. We were proud to be in uniform, but also knew we should try to keep a low profile, lest someone with RN or MD after their name ask us something we couldn't possibly know the first six months of nursing school. Donning my hideous striped dress, I would repeat a short mantra to myself: know your patient, write the perfect care plan.

The Spirit of Nursing | 33

Nursing training has changed dramatically since the days of white caps. It may be tempting to consider a discussion of uniforms and accessories superficial. With regards to nursing, it is not. The tools of the trade that nurses no longer carry hint at much larger changes in the profession, including the nurse's role in relationship to other providers of care.

Much has been said about what we wore on our heads, but we cannot forget the white clinic shoes nurses once wore. My first nursing shoes were the Pert model, made "For Women in White." They cost $10 a pair in 1975. I suppose they were worth it, since they promised to "do the job." In reality, they were a lot of work. Perts had to be polished and then buffed. Some of us learned that you could take the easy way out by applying the white polish then spraying them with a varnish.

We also replaced the shoelaces every two weeks. At that time the Head Nurse noticed if they were dirty; really, she seemed to notice everything. This shoe routine was done in addition to wearing support hose (even if you only weighed about a hundred pounds) under your uniform, which had to be starched and hemmed below the knee. Oh, and never forget the accompanying nursing pin, watch, and pen, all put in their own place, in the white plastic organizer, in the pocket of your uniform (not scrubs). But no stethoscope—those were for the doctors.

Forty years ago, nursing school students were required to wear a particular uniform and cap. They also needed a 3-colored pen, flashlight, bandage scissors and tape measure. The pen was for writing shift notes—daytime was blue, evening was green, and overnight was red. The bandage scissors were cleaned between patients with alcohol wipes, and the tape measure (to measure for abdominal binders, scultetus binder and anti-embolism stockings) was kept securely in your pocket.

Today, you could most likely work without a pen. Electronic medical records and electronic signatures have taken over. Our "in the pocket" bandage scissors were replaced years ago with sterile scissors, and we now have disposable tape measures for individual patient use. Notably, they are not being used for scultetus binders, for those have gone the way of the starched white pinafore. These are all positive changes, and so is the use of the stethoscope among nurses. When I was in nursing school, they were used primarily by physicians. RNs are now more responsible for auscultation of heart sounds, respiratory sounds, and their correlation to disease states than forty years ago.

We contribute to the patient's progress toward a health goal in most of the same ways, but I think our contributions may be more sophisticated. There are some things we have picked up, some things we have taken as our own, and others we have discarded, all for the benefit of the patient. And now, "in the pocket" means something totally different, for people with atrial fibrillation at least, it's "pill in the pocket."

During clinical, I lived to get the Kardex. It's funny, because now I live to get a computer that functions. The Kardex was a green cardstock paper, folded and formatted to contain patient information. But it was so much more than that; it had everything you needed to know. Because of the Kardex, even though nurses' notes were strictly written in black, green and red pen (Days, Evenings and Nights) you also needed to carry a pencil. Pen was forbidden in the Kardex. If you were crazy enough to forget, you had to hope you were also carrying whiteout, a product never seen now. In many cases, you would try to get to the Kardex early to do your Care Plan, preferably the night before.

In addition to passing examinations, there is the on-the-ground training and introduction to the profession that comes with the exciting and terrifying chaos of clinical. This is an important time in any nurse's career. No matter what has been learned up to that point (usually in a classroom) all nurses learn there is much, much more to come.

Nursing school is difficult, and it does not really prepare you for clinical rotations. I was eighteen years old tackling psychiatric nursing, surgical nursing, and OB / GYN nursing education. Overall, I thought psychiatric nursing clinical was the most challenging. I did this clinical rotation during the summer, and a particularly warm one at that. While I was assigned to several buildings at a State Hospital, we received a special visit from the governor. I was told in the morning that he would be arriving by helicopter that same day and would land in the medical center's field. In order to say hello to the patients, they'd be escorted out, leaving their units. This all sounded rather interesting, at least until preconference.

I learned that I would be responsible for keeping my two patients' hats on (because of the Thorazine) and to please ensure that they not roam. I was 5'2" and 105 pounds. My patients were schizophrenic, overweight, and anxious to escape. Though the building was usually locked, today the rules were lifted for the governor's visit. I did manage to keep my assignment of two patients safe. I also learned that it is nearly impossible to learn anything when you are terrified.

My first role as a new graduate was in the Intensive Care Unit. At the time, the general consensus was that three-year diploma graduates were more than prepared to take on this role. Maybe I should have been afraid, but I was not. As a graduate nurse, I had to work under the auspices of another RN until I passed my boards. In 1970, you took State Boards over two days but it took weeks to get the results. Those were long weeks. Eventually, there was scuttlebutt that the results were in. When I got home, my mother was holding the envelope. I asked her to open it. She read aloud: "Medical-Surgical: 4 0 0. Maternal Child Health: 4 0 0." I knew the minimum was 4 0 0 to pass. At this point, I am relieved, but also considering that I had just made it. I then realized that she was reading the passing grade instead of my achieved grade. Mine were much better.

I was 19 years old and embarking on my first day of clinical on the Obstetrical unit. I tried not to think too much about how different this was from medical-surgical. I was young, unmarried, and without children—and I was petrified when I walked in to hear several women screaming at the top of their lungs. All of the nurses on the unit were wearing giant pink and blue buttons on their uniforms that read: "OB nurses….at your cervix."

After 45 years of nursing, I remain humbled by my colleagues in obstetrical nursing.

Nurses have learned a lot about reducing fevers in patients over the years. We learned that many years before our nursing school education, nurses used phlebotomy; this was the preferred method before antipyretics. Generally, we were taught about conductive, convective, and evaporative methods of cooling as means of lowering body temperatures. Our main focus during my time in nursing school, however, was on alcohol baths.

In the 1970s, we were taught to use isopropyl alcohol on skin to quickly reduce a fever. I will never forget how one of my nursing student colleagues interpreted the process. After determining her patient needed the procedure, she read the policy and gathered the equipment. She had a small stainless bowl, sterile water, and about a thousand alcohol prep pads.

The instructor stopped before she had opened them all. I think she would have done much better with evaporated cooling, a few facecloths, and a fan. Today, we approach fevers differently; we do not require a thousand alcohol wipes.

I'll never forget my Cardiology instructor from nursing school. I often wonder if she proved the experts wrong, or if it wasn't really an emergency after all. Experts claim that cardiac arrest requires CPR, defibrillation, or at least Epinephrine. But I watched, wide-eyed, as my Cardiology instructor managed to scream someone out of cardiac arrest. She screamed his name as loud as I had ever heard anyone scream anything. He seemed to instantly wake up. I think I'll never know if it was sleep he woke up from or not. I am not sure it matters. It was clear he wasn't responding before the scream, and he was after.

I was given some memorable advice during one of my clinical rotations in 1980. The charge nurse told me, "don't ever be a noctor." "You won't make friends," she added. A noctor, it turns out, is a nurse who acts like a doctor. I found it troubling at the time because several of my professors were doctors. Now, I am proud of my many nursing colleagues who have achieved this distinction. We also call them Doctor, not noctor.

Patients have much to teach a novice nurse. While some patients are memorable for their pranks, others remain lodged in the memories of professionals many decades later for their courage.

As a junior nursing school student, it was an expectation that I rotate to the 3 p.m. to 11 p.m. shift at some point. When my turn came up, I was eager to do a great job. I remember being assigned to a male patient with the diagnosis of renal calculi. I spent the better part of an entire shift searching for his kidney stone in the filter. My diligence impressed the patient, and when the urologist rounded that evening, the patient told him how intent I was on finding the stone.

Later, the patient called me in to his room. I looked down to see the Holy Grail of stones in his urinal. The stone was so big it could not have possibly been passed by any human.

This particular urologist had a reputation for being a wonderful physician and unbeknownst to me, a prankster. It seems the urologist and the patient were in on the joke together. Earlier, the physician had gone out to get a parking lot stone to put into the urinal. Everyone had a good laugh, except for me...so much for my youthful enthusiasm.

Twenty-one years ago, I was a student in my first rotation in an extended care ward. There is one absolutely beautiful patient from that time that I will always remember. I remember the beauty of her face, her kindness, and her acceptance. This woman had a great personality and a love for life. Physically, she was a bodice with no extremities. Her ischemia had resulted in amputations, so she had no arms or legs. This meant that she lacked independence in all aspects of her life; she required help with toileting, eating, and dressing. She was lowered into a tub three times a week by a lift. She was fed by someone every day, three times a day. She could not even drink without it being directly in front of her, with straw in reach.

Over the past twenty-one years, I have often thought of her as someone who had every right to complain and be angry. But she didn't, and she wasn't. I found her demeanor to be as beautiful as she was. My first interaction with her was overwhelming to me as a student, but it taught me something important. I learned that even with the most comprehensive report or handoff, a nurse is never really prepared for the assessment they will find.

We called it "poor" in 1976. Now it would be termed "a socio-economic disadvantage" or a "health disparity." For this patient, I'm sure it didn't matter what we labeled it, she knew how it looked, smelled, and felt, not only physically but emotionally. She had several young children, so young that she was still breastfeeding the baby. I learned she was breastfeeding in spite of her cancer. This woman's tissues were necrotic; the cancer had engulfed her breast to a point that her skin was sloughing off. The main reason she presented to the emergency room was the odor. It was so intense that her family insisted.

I was young but couldn't imagine the only reason to seek medical help was because of the smell, especially after seeing her breast. I quickly learned, and although I'm not sure I understood, at the time, why. It was because of the baby, she explained. Now, the only way I can explain how it impacted me is this: relationships are hard to define. Not only person to person, but relationships between people and their beliefs and perceptions about themselves and their health. There are many nursing theories that help us to understand, guide our practice. But it was simple to her. There was nothing more important to this woman than feeding her baby. Not even her own life. It really didn't have anything to do with being poor.

At any age or stage in one's career, continuing one's education can be intimidating. As standards for higher education have increased within the profession, many nurses find themselves returning to post-secondary programs throughout their careers.

Though I was surprised by the differences in the courses I had taken for my bachelor's degree and my master's degree, I was not totally intimidated. Not until I took Advanced Physical Assessment. Two things frightened me about Advanced Physical Assessment: the otoscope and the speculum. I will start with the otoscope, but first, know that there was a lot of pressure to do well in this class, and for good reason. The amount of information needed to pass each examination was tremendous.

During eye, ear, nose, and throat (EENT) examinations, I was having difficulty visualizing and positioning the equipment. The harder I tried, the less I saw. The professor suggested I memorize the ear and eye anatomy, and then "use of the equipment would become natural." I did just that. I memorized. But when it was my turn to perform the examination for a grade, I must have taken the advice to "memorize" a bit too far. Looking in the eye, I confidently noted: "the cilia, the cone of light, the color, translucency of the tympanic membrane." I remember actually stating, "good visualization of the tympanic membrane." I was promptly stopped by the Professor and told to start over. Unfortunately, I repeated the same memorized version of a normal ear canal. I was looking in the eye.

The speculum was a different story. I was over the age of fifty, had delivered three ten-pound children, and I was sitting in a class with students in their twenties. No, I was not interested in "finding a partner" in the class so that I could do a vaginal exam on her and in return, have her "do one on me." So, I decide on the alternate option: performing the vaginal exam on the expert that had brought in to the university. I pay her cash. Many others in the class do, too. I wait in line for my turn to perform the exam on the so-called vaginal expert and I wonder about it the entire time I am waiting. I do not know what makes one a vaginal expert, but I did pass Advanced Physical Assessment.

In the end, a nurse receives an education in his or her profession in many ways: in the classroom, the clinical setting, and often, through years of working with colleagues. Role models may come in many forms, but what is most important is that nurses look out for one another.

As a young female desperately trying to find her footing, I was juggling my life as a nursing student, working full-time to pay for school, and trying to meet family obligations, all at once. I was overwhelmed, and haunted by the fact that I had previously been told that I could not be a good nurse because of my background. I started to miss class and had difficulty focusing. My studies were lacking, and I was struggling.

During this time, one of my professors (who regularly spoke with and checked in on all students) noticed what I was going through. One day, she told me that I needed to go to the library, away from my peers, to gather my thoughts and study. She then told me that there was more to talk about, so we met in her office the following day. When she asked me why I wanted to be a nurse, I stopped short. I told her plainly that I had never imagined being anything but a nurse. Caring for others made me feel like I could make a difference. She explained that "a caring heart and a desire to heal" was exactly what every nurse needed.

This professor then tasked me with ranking my obligations and immediate needs. I quickly recognized that none of my other obligations could be fulfilled if I did not care for myself and make nursing school my highest priority. This faculty member frequently checked in with me and became a much-needed source of support and guidance. It has been years since I graduated and yet I still hear from her. She is always eager to hear about my accomplishments and proud of my chosen path. I recognize that this type of person is a treasure that many people do not get to find. I am thankful that she recognized where I was and helped me acknowledge where I needed to be. I am appreciative for the support I had, and in return, I continuously try to help the nursing students and new graduates who, like me, find themselves at a crossroad. I also remember that "a caring heart and a desire to heal" can be communicated with an empathetic smile or therapeutic touch. This nursing professor will always be my guardian angel. Her example guides me as I try to be a supportive mentor, something I learned from her.

Every nursing program has its assets, and in spite of the many years we have tried to decide what degree is best for patient outcomes, I still believe that caring and insight are the most important attributes you can have and learn as a nurse. The truth is that I was taught the technical aspects of nursing in school. But I always knew that the most important attribute—being a caring nurse—would not be on any exam or even the NCLEX. After graduating, I learned quickly that my new colleagues, no matter what degree they achieved, all had both, the technical and the caring. That's how I learned from the best.

Being a Nurse is a title that I hold with abundant pride, integrity, and honor. For the past 21 years, I have justly embraced the role and practice of nursing and have never once regretted my decision to choose it as my lifelong profession. I pursued my education continuously since kindergarten. I have changed my career goals a few times, but 21 years ago, I was able to get the opportunity to finally reach my longtime dream of becoming a nurse. I have since earned a master's degree in healthcare. As I reached each milestone, my understanding of the importance of my role and the responsibilities of a nurse have evolved. I am in awe of the ever-changing healthcare climate. Through it all, there is one person who has never altered her outlook or prospects for the nursing profession. She has exuded the true spirit of nursing.

Throughout my career, some have disrespected, abused, mocked, interrogated, and challenged the profession of nursing. Others have admired and respected it. Through all of these trials and tribulations in the day of a nurse, and the innumerable encounters of opinions, demands and commands, I have never lost my true hunger to remain a dedicated nurse and to advocate for those in my care. I remain a dedicated, passionate, and compassionate nurse. I have never deviated from the basic understanding of the utmost importance of my role in caring for others. More than ever, I appreciate the compassion necessary to care for patients and loved ones. This is the true reason I aspired to become a nurse in the first place, along with the help, guidance, and admiration I have for my mentor. She is the best role model of our profession I personally have ever encountered.

Throughout my career, I have worked in many different roles. I have met many people in the healthcare profession. But she stands out. She has been my true inspiration since the day I had the privilege and the opportunity to be taught and mentored by her. I have been inspired by her; she has become a friend. I have never ceased to be totally mesmerized by her efforts. I continue to watch her exemplify the value of nursing and its profession. She has embodied what the commitment of being a nurse means. I owe my level of understanding, appreciation, and continued commitment to her.

Chapter Three

A Patient I'll Never Forget

Kristine Batty, Patti Bonzagni,
Jeannine Borozny, Becky Carley,
Linda Del Vecchio-Gilbert, Bob Desrosiers,
Pam DiMascio, Donna Dupuis, Lucille Ferrer,
Leiah Gallagher, Marla Goulart, Donna Horrocks,
Lisa Johnson, Elaine Joyal, Rachel Jones,
Rebecca Jones, Mary Lavin, Shelley MacDonald,
Alisha Mal, Michelle Mallon, Colleen Moynihan,
Deb Myers, Stacie Nunziato, Kathy O'Connell,
Angela Quarters, Deb Quirk, Liz Raposa,
Cathy Schwartz, Linda Tierney, Karen Treloar,
Cindy Votto, Ginny Wilcox, Karen Zarlenga

"They may forget your name, but they will never forget how you made them feel."

Maya Angelou

What does it mean to care for another human being? All nurses know that some elements of what they do have been around for millennia. They also acknowledge that changes in practice have rapidly altered their work even within one lifetime. This is part of the difficulty with describing what a nurse actually does. They take on both mundane tasks and extraordinary challenges every single day in clinical practice. They watch as babies take their first breaths. They are also there as older adults and unfortunately, sometimes much younger people take their last.

Nurses are there for the big and small tragedies and triumphs that can occur in between life and death. After reviewing their countless hours of clinical practice, the contributors to this chapter have chosen to reflect on select, important moments in their careers. While some stories are about high points, others relate equally important lows. All nurses have had moments of questioning, doubt, fear, or anxiety. Those days are thankfully often balanced out with the tremendous feeling of truly reaching out and caring for someone else. Patients, after all, are more than an assignment.

Many nurses have experienced the burden and privilege of being with patients as they die. As a result, quite a few stories in this chapter relate those moments. Those who do not make it can often be among the most memorable in a nurse's career. Looking back on the care they have given, some nurses think of the patients for whom they were able to make all the difference, saving them from death, at least for the time being. For others, there is the peace of knowing that they were able to make an end-of-life transition more merciful.

The connection between nurse and patient is like nothing else. In caring for another person, a nurse must be aware of a million small details. They must also never lose sight of the whole person. Though so much of healthcare can be thought of in empirical terms, that is not the only way to see nursing. In this profession, there is also what some call "the gentle art of caring," that harder to locate skill that is no less essential to practice. The highs and lows of nursing can often be difficult to communicate to those outside of the profession—this is part of that "knowing" only those who have worked as nurses share. We could say it is indescribable, but we have done our best to convey what it has meant to us.

The first stories in this chapter begin with life itself: pregnancy, childbirth, and infancy. Caring for those who are anticipating childbirth and/or extremely vulnerable babies comes with particular challenges, though the rewards are just as great.

The year was around 1974. The patient was a 30-year-old woman admitted in her last trimester with vaginal bleeding. Back then, a patient could stay in the hospital for weeks without question. Nurses could be assigned to the same patients for weeks, too. Toward the end of her stay, this patient delivered a beautiful baby girl. I was both surprised and honored when she named the baby after me. I was able to care for this patient postpartum, and I was grateful for that. We spent a lot of time talking about how she was going to be able to love this child conceived of rape. I hoped and prayed that she would always look at her daughter the same way she did that day she was born. I still think of that baby and mother, and it's not just because of her name.

It was 1968 and I was a student nurse on a three-month OB / GYN rotation. Each of us had been assigned a patient from the community to follow through the birthing process, and our clinicals involved journaling. My patient was complicated. Along with the responsibility of giving birth alone, she was worried about her husband serving in Vietnam. I spent a lot of time with her. Since I did not have a car, I had to rely on my parents to get to my clinicals. My biggest fear was that I would miss the birth. I didn't miss it, though. I was with her throughout the birth, holding her hand. The baby was a perfect girl. Much to my surprise, the first time my patient saw her new baby girl, she called her by my name. I'll never forget either of them.

I remember being at a function with friends and a woman came up to me and asked if I was a nurse. When I replied yes, she said "I knew it." She told me she would never forget my eyes or voice. She asked if I recalled taking a ride from a hospital to transfer a patient in crisis. I confirmed that I did. She pointed out a tall slender teen and stated "this is the child I later delivered following our ambulance ride." She continued, "It was the warmth of your eyes, the gentleness in your assuring voice, and the touch of holding your hand, that provided me great comfort during my transfer to the other hospital, feeling comfort that myself and baby would be safe."

Many years ago, I had the pleasure of caring for a 4-month-old baby boy during my pediatric rotation as a student nurse. The admitting diagnosis was bronchiolitis. This was the cause of his hospital admission, but it was not his only problem. This boy had multiple congenital abnormalities leading to complex care needs. Weighing about 7 pounds, this baby had a long, pointed tongue. He demonstrated lizard-like actions and had a strange palmar deviation. He was unable to support his head and had a severe diaper rash. In the three days he was hospitalized, he was being cared for by strangers. This poor, helpless little guy stole my heart. He required a lot of attention but I was more than happy to provide it.

Of everything I did to help this child, I think the most important thing I could provide was tender care. I cuddled him, fed him, and sang to him. He would smile, coo, and babble. I couldn't help but wonder what the future would hold for him and how many obstacles he would face. I often still think of him. He would be an adult today if he did in fact survive. He will never know who I am or that I helped care for him. He will also never know what a joy it was for me or how he touched my life.

Outside of obstetrics, most nurses do not meet their patients on the first day of their lives. They are entering an unknown chapter in a longer story. Sometimes, unfortunately, that meeting can happen in an early chapter. Many caregivers acutely remember their encounters with especially young patients, in part because their traumas can seem especially poignant.

On the first day of my pediatric clinical rotation in my junior year of nursing school, I met a patient I will never forget. I was placed at an inner-city elementary school that had a doctor's office in the building. I was waiting for another patient to come into the office when a herd of adults suddenly came storming in. Something seemed to be happening. A nurse asked me to sit down and watch a little boy for a few minutes. I went with this child into another room and we started to color with crayons. From the conversation I made with him, it seemed to me that he was a happy little boy who just liked to color.

Moments later, the nurse pulled me aside to inform me as to what had happened. Earlier that day, this boy had tried to kill himself during class. He took pens and attempted to suck out the ink so he could "be with someone he loved, in heaven." The nurse, teacher, social worker, and principal decided that it was best that he be picked up from school. After much discussion with him, I assessed that he was not as happy as he appeared to be. He did not feel as though he had true friends; he was being bullied. This little boy had a tough life. His story really touched me. I tried to follow up the next week at clinical. I was able to talk to him again. I was relieved. From what the child told me, he had not tried to hurt himself again. For the rest of the clinical rotation, I periodically checked up on him. Self-harm is a serious matter. I still wonder about the follow up for this little boy. Would it be enough? I thought he would stay in my mind for a long time and he has.

I will never forget the very young patient I took care of who was impaled while climbing a tree. He lost an eye and had extensive orbital damage, which resulted in neurological problems. His hospitalization led to a tracheostomy, which he constantly tried to take out or cough out. It was a struggle to maintain for both the patient and the staff.

We were always aware of needing that sterile, metal spare tracheostomy taped to the headboard. I vividly remember working the night shift, constantly worried about that metal tracheostomy tube; I'm also acutely aware that this patient most likely spent a majority of the night shift worried about breathing through the new hole in his throat. I hope he was not too afraid.

Some nurses recall particular patients not so much for what they endured but because they were hospitalized in the prime of their lives. In some instances, it can be hard to imagine these people outside of the hospital. Yet something as simple as a photograph or poster can conjure a whole other life, creating a starting point for nurse and patient to bond.

I once had a patient who was a gifted lover of music. Tragically, a spinal cord injury had left this young man a quadriplegic. In the hospital room, Beethoven and Bach posters hung over his bed. Visitors spoke about him in glowing terms; he was "a great teacher," an "admirable man," someone "intelligent and gifted." When I met him, he had recovered enough to be considered eligible for rehabilitation care. He still had his tracheostomy, so he often attempted to speak but it was unintelligible. This made him frustrated. He was angry at his inability to communicate. His arms and legs would spasm and become outstretched, shaking—a reminder he had no control.

This patient also had difficulties with feeding and aspirating. I had trouble feeding him. During his hospital stay, we would often have lunch together. One particular day, I accidently took a sip of his drink instead of my own. I felt horrible, but he found a lot of humor in it. His laughter was mixed with hissing and sneezing, but you knew he was very amused. I went from feeling horrible to feeling embarrassed to happy. He had found humor again. He eventually found ways to communicate through typing with a pencil in his mouth. Occupational Therapy enhanced this by creating a metal device for his arm, one with some movement and feeling. He always had a lot to say, and he had many requests and many stories. We always wanted to listen. His group of caregivers was hardworking; we worked together to care for him and to respect him. None of us ever wanted to disappoint him. There were days we didn't have enough staff to get him out of bed, or back to bed in the evening. One of us would always return to the hospital to do it, long after we had gone home. I will never forget him.

In the picture she was beautiful. Smiling with a cocktail in hand, she was so full of life. In the bed where she lay critically ill, she was frail. This patient had been intubated, her vital signs were threatening, and she had a multitude of infusions. Her husband sat with his chair right up against the bed, in front of the ventilator. It was the same as the day before and the day before that. Today, however, he had brought the picture. "This is what she's supposed to look like," he said. This photograph served as a subtle reminder that we don't just support people's ventilator settings and adjust hemodynamics. As nurses, we support families and their hopes for a life that is different from what is happening to them—a life the way it should be.

Sometimes humor is necessary, even in the darkest moments. It may not seem appropriate, but often in recovery, in the moment you realize someone just might live, it comes out. It makes for a defining moment and as a nurse, you recognize it right away. This moment might be when a patient is no longer pyretic or when the norepinephrine gets the mean arterial pressure to greater than 70. Or, it can be when the patient is able to get out of bed for the first time. "Getting out of bed" is a term we use lightly, at times. It's not often with the patient's own strength this happens, in fact, it's often they don't have any strength. But we instinctively know why it's an important step. Families sometimes have a different way of articulating it.

With this patient, the moment happened on Easter morning. After days of recovering from surgeries, intubation, complications, and infection, we got the patient out of bed for the first time. To be clear, she did not get out of bed, we got her out of bed. Her husband came to visit right after. His first comment came quickly: "Lazarus has risen." It was a palpable moment for everyone. She was eventually discharged. She left with scars from a critical illness she will never forget. We imagine she is grateful for her recovery—we know that her husband was. For years, we would receive an Easter delivery, a fruit basket, from him and "Lazarus." We understood the reference. We have been witness to resurrection many times.

I had always dreamed of "hanging out my own shingle" and using my knowledge to help people with healthcare problems. Little did I know that this would lead me to a degree as an Advanced Practice Nurse. I have had many opportunities in APRN positions to provide healthcare to people needing a variety of interventions, from motivational interviewing to diagnostic studies. What I have loved most is listening to people to understand what they really need. I know this has made a difference to me and many people I have met, such as the patient I convinced to go for a screening colonoscopy who found her cancer at Stage I.

Another "neighborhood nurse" intervention would help my good friend. She was admitted to the ICU with sepsis after an infection of her hip replacement. She was non-responsive and it seemed that there was little hope for her survival. When I went to visit her, I was accompanied by another friend. We decided it was very important for the nursing staff to know what a smart, wonderful, caring person she was. As we performed reiki over her, we talked to her about how important she was to us. We left hoping we would get to see her again. My good friend survived to tell how she heard every word we said. Good thing it was all positive. I love every aspect of the nurse practitioner role and have continued my work as the "neighborhood nurse." I'm proud to be a one-woman tele-health operation. There are so many pictures of body parts and rashes on my phone; this unusual collection is paired with texts full of medical questions. Little did I know.

Nurses strive to care and connect. Sometimes, they realize long after the fact that perhaps they could not have known the exact right thing to do or say.

It was Christmas Day and I was at second lunch (12:00 p.m.). I never thought I would get second lunch, especially on Christmas Day. But this was not the most improbable thing—it was the man walking toward me. There was a time when I thought I would never see this man walk again. He had spent weeks recovering from a serious injury. He had fallen while rock climbing; that injury was complicated by a pre-existing bone disease. The bone disease didn't stop him from having a family, but it did make recovering from this injury more challenging.

Being in healthcare himself, this man understood everything. He recovered from the shock and we stabilized him. Eventually he was transferred for restorative care and his fractures healed. On his way from rehabilitation to skilled nursing, he visited intensive care. He still looked so angry. He never looked afraid or sad, just angry. It was as if he felt that something had been taken away from him. I think it was because he knew. Being in healthcare, he knew the trajectory of his disease and his injury, including the possible future injuries. But today, during second lunch, I saw a man who was no longer angry. He walked toward me, family in tow, with a new look and fresh flowers in hand. Getting second lunch on Christmas day paled in comparison to this.

In the early 1980s, I decided to become a nurse practitioner. My first clinical experience was in a city hospital. During that time, I cared for many patients who were indigent. One such patient that I will never forget was in the process of a transition. While seeking housing at a shelter, they had been upset by the idea of showering and changing in view of females. This did not match with their gender identity, yet they were also not allowed at the men's shelter. This person had many medical issues, and we were able to treat those. But we did little to improve the real issue in his life, as he saw it. I will never forget this patient that I failed to help. I was completely unprepared to assist this patient with their situation.

There are some patients that nurses are inclined to remember because of their difficulties they presented to the staff. Though patients are incredibly vulnerable, those who care for them also face their own dangers. As nurses well know, their daily practice may include long stretches of banal tasks, but these days are punctuated with situations that range from mildly frustrating to deeply frightening.

My first year in an ICU was pure joy. I learned constantly from the best mentors and wonderful friends. I have so many patients that I still remember after more than four decades. It seems funny, in a way, how you remember them—it's a triad, really: name, diagnosis, room. I suppose this is part of being a nurse.

As a new graduate, I was very serious about patient education. I was also very naïve. I was assigned to a patient with COPD. He had multiple admissions for exacerbation. I dismissed my colleagues' advice that education about stopping smoking was not effective on him. I needed to try. Unfortunately, after one half hour of discussing the effects of smoking he pulled out the Lucky Strikes from under his chair and lit up.

On another occasion, I had a patient who was admitted with R / O Psyche. That was it; this was an acceptable diagnosis at the time. I went to her room and she wasn't there. I imagined the worst. I found her in another patient's room about to adjust the Lidocaine drip. Most of the patients on the cardiac unit had a Lidocaine drip. No pump, just the drip waiting to be drip calculated, but preferably by the RN.

Two years after I graduated, I changed jobs from a small, non-teaching ICU to a teaching institution. There is one night shift in particular that I remember. I was assigned to a patient who was exhibiting violent behavior, perhaps related to ingestion. I heard a crash from the nurse's station and learned he had broken from his restraints. This patient was naked and had pieces of glass from his broken IV bottle in hand. He grabbed me, pulled me toward him, and threatened to hurt me with the glass. An intern assigned to the ICU, who was slight, attempted to help but he was no match. Once the police arrived, we were safe. Most people would not imagine that a nurse's role is sometimes this dangerous.

The truth is that most nurses have at least been verbally threatened. It does not change our love for the patients but it forces us to realize how fortunate, but vulnerable, we are.

It was three months after I graduated from nursing school. I may have been a little overzealous when I volunteered to care for several young men who had been burned in a fire at the local correctional facility. I had never heard some of the words that came out of their mouths, even though I had three brothers. Over the next two months, I learned to care for burn victims. I also learned a lot about how to be a better nurse. Caring for these men, I came to understand that judging someone based on their words is a terrible thing. It was easy to be judgmental, but that would mean seeing my patient through their limits instead of their potential. I never wanted to be on the wrong side of that equation. Looking back on it now, there were times when I was tested. I tried to remember how fortunate I was not to have been burned, or to have been addicted to alcohol or drugs. Eventually the boys healed. Their skin became a little bit tougher, and mine did, too.

Good listeners make for good nurses. While not all patients are able to communicate in a traditional sense, a nurse has to find a way to listen and respond to the sometimes- unspoken needs of those they care for. As these stories suggest, everyone needs to be heard.

I remember a client that had an important message for me. He was admitted to the unit in the room at the very end of the hallway. I remember learning that this gentleman in his sixties had been married for more than 40 years. His wife was so involved in his care—so loving and attentive. She never left him. One evening he and his wife were having an argument. She left hurriedly, racing to the elevator. That night her husband unexpectedly died. Unfortunately, she was on her way back into the unit to see him, when the physician saw her and had to break the news. I have never heard anyone cry so hard.

She later explained that throughout their 40-year marriage they almost never fought. If they did, they would not leave each other until they had made up. She cried so hard about not ever being able to make up with him. She would not have the opportunity. The profession of nursing is not just a rewarding career but a career full of life lessons. I now do not go to bed angry or leave angry. I try to remember to say I love you. We never know when we will see a loved one again.

My first job was working the third shift on a 30-bed medical-surgical unit in a teaching hospital. I was so fortunate because the charge nurse (the only other full-time nurse on the shift) had over 20 years of experience and became my mentor. On good nights, there were also two aides to help us. The first year was a period of intense learning and confidence building. I learned to see in the dark, to comfort patients who could not sleep, read patient's medical records, and to call for help when needed. Every patient was a different puzzle. What worked for one did not always help another. I eventually left the night shift after realizing that I was nervous being around too many people at a shopping mall during the holidays. When I got on the day shift (with rotations to nights and evenings) I faced other challenges. There were so many people and so much going on.

Thankfully, rounding with the physicians and other members of the health care team reinforced my self-confidence and role as a patient advocate. Being sick and in the hospital was scary and not where most people wanted to be. I always thought we need to treat our patients as if they were our own families, because someday they will be. I always tried to ask my patients to tell me about themselves, what they liked to do, what they didn't like to do, and what they were looking forward to. Each has their own story and was special in their own way.

It was a typical morning on the medical surgical floor. I was a new nurse. My patient was down at the end of the long hall. I reviewed his history: RUE embolectomy, diabetes, and a stroke. I also looked at his vitals, blood sugar, labs, and orders—everything looked good. I had my day all planned. With my supplies, I walked down the hall, knocking to enter his room. It was about 8 : 00 a.m. I said good morning and introduced myself, but all I heard was "Ko-Di-Ko."

In the bed, I saw a man around 60-years-old who appeared older than his age. He was bald and toothless. He was also a bilateral above the knee amputee. His left arm was paralyzed and his upper right extremity was immobilized, elevated in a 45-degree IV pole sling. As I do my initial assessment, offering him a drink and feeding him breakfast, I hear him say "Ko-Di-Ko." I learn that due to aphasia, he can only utter this one phrase. It is all he can say to communicate everything to everyone. He is frustrated and upset; overwhelmed, his face turns red. I explain that he is in a hospital and has had surgery. I also explain the reason his arm has been immobilized and how important it is for recovery despite how inconvenient it seems. He looks at me as if I am crazy. Of course, he knew all that. I talk to him some more, asking him questions along the way. All he could do was nod yes and no and say "Ko-Di-Ko."

Through trial and error, we gradually began to understand each other. He calmed down, started to accept my care, and even trusted me. He guided me through every medication, motion of the wash cloth, movement of the pillow, placement of his sheet, positioning of the blanket, and height adjustment of the bed. I could see that underneath this very helpless man was an independent person who had been stripped of all control. But he was determined to maintain as much independence as possible. By the time we got through our routine, it was 9 : 45 AM. The patient smiled and said "Ko-Di-Ko" again, this time in a soft and gentle tone. A tear ran down his cheek. I hugged him and watched him doze off for a nap.

I walked out of his room exhausted but very satisfied that I had been able to help him. I learned such a valuable lesson from this patient: humility. He taught me to be thankful for little things. I have two legs that I can walk on, two arms I can move, and a voice to speak with. So, when things are not going well, I try not to feel sorry for myself. I learned that it can always be worse, and that strength comes from within. Over the past forty years, I have often thought about this man who I affectionately remember as "Ko-Di-Ko." He gave me so much more than I gave him.

Many clients have taught me lessons. I will always remember the young woman in her twenties who was diagnosed with a form of ALS. She had two young children and a devoted husband who would leave his job to care for her. Her prognosis was poor; she was only given about a year to live. She was admitted many times with different complications from her disease. Her goal was to see her daughter graduate from high school. She would have to live more than the year she was given. She did not see her dream come true.

With all her admissions and physical deteriorations throughout the years she was always upbeat and smiling. We never know what is in our path of life, but we must keep our eye on our goals. Perhaps the lesson is not so much to complete the goal or see the dream come true, especially if you are so unfortunate as she was. It's a cliché but maybe our dreams are in the minutes instead of months and years. One thing I am sure of, she never disappointed her daughter or husband. They were proud of the way she fought.

My patient was admitted about 9 : 30 at night. Her family came in with her, and followed her from the emergency room. I sensed she was putting on a brave face for them. I settled her in and her family left for the evening. At about 11: 30 p.m. I heard screaming and sobbing coming from her room. "I am going to die tonight, call my family back, now!"

I assessed all of her vital signs, sat with her, and assessed her physically. I found no change. I tried to reassure her. By the time I left her room she was more relaxed. I remember saying it was going to be OK. I went to check on her about 15 minutes after that. That's when I heard it. You learn about the pattern of it, but it's unmistakable when you hear it. It is called agonal breathing. We coded her for thirty-five minutes. It was determined to be a pulmonary embolism. I will never forget her face. I will never tell a patient "it's going to be ok." Although the final diagnosis was pulmonary embolism, I believe I failed this patient. I don't believe I failed to give her the physical, medicinal nursing care she deserved. I believe I failed to listen.

I vividly recall my feelings of inadequacy when I was assigned one of those patients with the tattoos. I used to think this type of care deserved a special orientation, because none of us were sure of the rules. Personally, I only knew that my father refused to talk about it. My only knowledge was what I had learned in high school, and although the war had ended thirty years earlier, I had not been given enough information to know what was appropriate.

Looking at their arms, I wondered if I should ask. I know I wanted to. But I didn't dare. I was afraid; it would be insensitive; the question might be misinterpreted. They were all so strong. No matter what diagnosis they received, no matter how much suffering they endured, they all reacted the same way. With strength, endurance, and a fierce will. I had never seen anything like this as a young nurse.

I did not care for many Holocaust survivors, the patients with tattoos. But I cared for enough to know their attributes and to decide that no diagnosis, no amount of painful procedures, tests or interventions would ever compare. I often think about this small cohort of patients with such important needs. I wonder if I may have failed to meet those needs. I knew my practice needed to incorporate more understanding, more sensitivity. But I may have failed to provide it. As a nurse, you often think back to the patients you have cared for, very often questioning if you did the right thing. It is not often whether you gave the right medication at the right time, it's more of a humanitarian question that you ask yourself. Decades later, I still wonder about these patients. Did I compromise? Perhaps I did. I didn't ask these patients what they needed. They never told. Perhaps not talking about it is how they survived. I will never forget those tattoos. They have probably forgotten me, but I know there is much more they cannot.

Compassionate care is always the high standard for nurses. Sometimes, however, practitioners may feel as though they have fallen short. Other times, nurses will know that they give the best care possible for a particular patient, which in time may prove to be a small comfort.

I remember a young mother who sustained a sudden cardiac arrest. Her family wanted to donate her organs so others may have the chance to live. This type of nursing took the highest level of support, compassion, and caring.

Within the first six months of becoming an oncology nurse I met one compassionate man. It was while caring for a patient who was actively dying, but alone. He had no family and no visitors. Every chance I got I would spend a few minutes with him, but it may not have been enough... at least in the eyes of my other patient, a young man who was only 36 at the time.

During one of my visits, I found this man sitting with the patient who was at the end of his life, holding his hand. I know it comforted him because I could see it. Within a short time, the patient died peacefully. The man with all of the compassion, who had been holding his hand, was young, healthy looking, and married with a six-year-old son. He had received the diagnosis of anxiety after complaining of abdominal pain. But after more diagnostics, it became advanced gastric cancer; his prognosis was three months. This caring, compassionate young man was discharged to prepare for his own death.

A few months later at the end of his life he was readmitted. He was still so strong. He did not shed tears for his life that was being cut so short but was focused on preparing his family for life without him. He shared the details of this dying process with me so I could help others. Every night during his last two weeks I would sit with him while he shared his thoughts, feelings, and perceptions of what was happening to his body. I learned so much about life and death from him and have used this knowledge to help and comfort others during my career. I felt fortunate to be with him, his wife, and son when he left this world. A religious man, he was looking forward to the next adventure and catching up with the patient he had comforted. I am such a better nurse for all he taught me.

This patient kept me and my colleagues so busy that we literally named a weekend after him. The "Edward" weekend. A 55-year-old gentleman exhibiting what was most likely a manic episode, this man spent several days and nights circling our rectangular unit. He wasn't pacing or walking. No, he was running, sprinting like Tom Hanks in *Forrest Gump*, suitcase in hand. We gave him things to eat and drink as he squared the corners on the unit. We locked the doors. Still, he continued to run and circle around the nurses' station about every two minutes. At the end of the weekend, he was transferred to a state hospital. To this day, when I correspond with colleagues that I worked with at that time, they'll reminisce about that Edward weekend. Some years later I received an envelope in the mail with this man's obituary—no note, just the death notice.

When I think back, I don't really understand why we didn't do more for him, or could we have? All I kept thinking that day was: he's assigned to me. He's in my care. These patients are human beings assigned to be in your care. "In your care" means many different things. To me it means always remembering that they should not be in pain and they should not suffer. It also means treating all patients with the same respect that you would give your loved ones. I know that I did respect this man who continuously circled the unit with his suitcase. Now, I know that we would treat this man differently in terms in medical care. But I know that we did our best, at the time, to show him compassion.

The patient I can't forget was adamant. "Only the redhead can put my IV in," she said, and she meant it. It's actually my fault. Not the red hair—I had always wanted it and at age fifty, I made it happen. The part I do take the blame for is this patient only wanting "the redhead." She refused to have anyone else insert her IV. At first, she had refused me, too. That was until we talked about being redheads, discussing the fact that my red hair came from a box labeled L'Oréal 5R, hers from the Clairol # 6. This redhead talk broke the tension. It was then that I promised her I could get the IV in with one try. "It's my specialty," I told her. "Most redheads don't even have to try to be good at things," I continued. She laughed, let me try and I got it in.

End of story, or so I thought. Every time the IV had to be replaced, I was paged. Every time she just wanted to chat, I was paged. She learned how to do it from her room phone and her own cell phone. It wasn't a burden. It was actually an honor to think I won this patient over with a box of L'Oréal 5R. This patient was eventually discharged but readmitted several times as her condition declined. COPD sometimes has a predictable decline over a period of months. She was fearful, because instinctively she knew the trajectory, even though no one may have told her, exactly.

As a nurse, I was more than aware that she knew. That was why she kept my beeper number, even when she was discharged. Every time she was readmitted, I was paged. Every time she paged me, I responded. It was the red hair. She died a few months later.

I know I've used this gift before. The gift of influence. The ability to influence a patient to go in a direction they didn't want to go in. I've used it many times in thirty years. At times, patients refuse to go in the direction we advocate. They have the right. I know how important autonomy is, that freedom that is all yours and that no one can take away, especially when you need it the most. We accept and honor this as part of our professionalism; it is, simply part of being human and having empathy. I also believe, personally, that we can't choose everything in our lives, but sometimes we can make some our own destiny—with a little help from L'Oréal, or Clairol.

While I was a student some forty years ago, I worked as a nursing assistant at a local hospital. One of the patients that I will always remember was a middle-aged woman who was hit by a motor vehicle while she was in the crosswalk. She sustained trauma to both lower extremities. This patient ultimately lost both her legs. At the time, we did not have the multimodal pain management that exists now. As she underwent a transmetatarsal amputation, followed by a below knee amputation, and ultimately an above the knee amputation, this woman suffered greatly.

I can still vividly recall her rocking in the bed, cradling her amputated limb, and sobbing about the unbearable pain in her foot. I tried to understand what she was telling me and what I was seeing. As a young nursing student, I had read about phantom pain. Some believed it was a psychosomatic response to tissue loss. I was overwhelmed with the inadequacy of this explanation as I tried to ease the suffering of this incredibly valiant woman.

When the toes of the remaining leg began to discolor and the surgeons spoke of another transmetatarsal amputation, she refused. She insisted they take the whole leg as she could not bear to repeat the experience she just had. I learned so many things from this patient. I learned to really listen to what a patient tells you they are experiencing. Caring for this woman made me question my ideas, my knowledge, my attitudes about patient needs, and my nursing practice. There is always new science, technology, and information to assist us in becoming practitioners if we remain open to it. We have to question previously held assumptions and truly listen.

Toxic shock syndrome was one of the most feared complications from a bacterial infection in the 1980s. I remember caring for more than one patient who was seriously ill from it. There was a lot of speculation at the time as to the culprit, but for the patients who had it, it didn't really matter. They just wanted to survive it. Fever, shock, skin peeling and fasciitis, as well as emboli that caused extremities to become necrotic—this was the scenario for more than one of our patients.

Even those who survived due to expert care faced trauma-induced amputations, disabilities, and psychologiucal effects we had difficulty treating. One patient who survived multiple surgeries and amputations was struggling to readjust. We just could not get her to eat, even though her physical condition no longer warranted any restrictions. So, we tried something different: we promised her hot wieners (her favorite) and she promised to eat them. The next night, the whole floor, and perhaps even the whole hospital, was ripe with the smell of four hot wieners done up "all the way," with meat, onions, and so on. We all agreed the smell was worth it. Why can't your first meal after weeks of parenteral nutrition be four "all the way?"

I was asked to represent my community hospital in a recruitment video. The question I needed to answer was: "What makes this hospital a community hospital?" I immediately thought about a patient I took care of while working in one. For years I exercised by walking through a small village near my home. I would wave when I saw familiar faces, chatting with fellow walkers and runners. Then, one of those faces was in front of me one morning, waiting for a procedure. She had been running and had an event causing her to be admitted to the hospital. We chatted for a bit and exchanged introductions. She was obviously very nervous and I tried to reassure her that I would be with her during and after the procedure. The procedure went well, she received excellent news.

Although I have changed my walking route, I often go to the same village for other entertainment. I was attending a summer concert one evening and I spotted her sitting with friends. I approached her. Not only as a "walker" but as her nurse. She hugged me. She had tears in her eyes. I asked her…… "I don't know if you remember me……" I never expected to hear, "I will never forget you." To me, it was a routine procedure. We perform them every day. But not on her. That day it mattered that I was there. It mattered she was in my community hospital.

A nurses' career is filled with thousands of stories about caring for individuals. There are also many chapters dedicated to particular diagnoses or clinical issues, methods of care, and other aspects of practice.

My story is not about one patient in particular but a diagnosis. I have always had a special compassion for patients with obesity. Over the twenty years I have been a nurse, the prevalence of obesity has increased along with the complications of type 2 diabetes and hypertension. In the past five years, it has been actually recognized as a disease. Yet I am not sure that all of my colleagues in nursing and medicine embrace this. Recognizing that it is a disease has not helped the stigma.

Compared to other diagnoses, obesity continues to have more of a negative connotation. I think being a bedside nurse and doing the actual physical care on patients with this disability has made a difference. This experience has led me to believe that the idea of dignity can become foreign to someone who is unable to feel fresh, clean, and attractive to others. I don't think any aspect of their life is without trial. Retail stores, airlines, and movie theatres are all designed to be inaccessible to them. I have cared for patients who are morbidly obese (with diseases such as Prader-Willi and hyperphagia) who spend enormous amounts of energy attempting to get more to eat. It must be so difficult to live knowing you can't quit what is killing you.

Nurses are taught that adult respiratory distress syndrome, or ARDS, was once called Da Nang lung because it was recognized in the battlefield during the war in Vietnam. An ICU nurse knows that this disease is still a kind of battlefield for the patient. It is a "spectrum of disease." Within hours of diagnosis, the patient may need to be sedated, mechanically ventilated, and neuromuscular-blocked. That is the easy part, though— not for the patient, but for the nurse. Experience and education gave me the expertise to titrate sedation, alleviate the patient's pain, and control breathing. The hardest and most important aspect of a patient's recovery is remembering that there is a human being inside that body, the one that can't move, speak or cry.

The patient I will never forget was sedated, paralyzed, ventilated and put in a prone position in an effort to oxygenate his lungs. Oxygenation was not a problem a few hours earlier; that's how quickly it happens. That is the paradox of ARDS. During the month this patient fought to survive, I focused on the importance of conversation. I would talk about what day it was, what time it was, who I was, and where he was. He didn't move his own body, or breathe for himself for almost a month. But while you are waiting for the inflammation to subside, there's work to do. Part of a nurse's work involves the relationship he/she builds with that human being in the bed. This is just as critical as the Ativan drip.

After his recovery, this particular patient came back to the ICU. This was weeks after he underwent rehabilitation for the debilitation caused by ARDS. Turning to me, he said, "You're MY nurse." He continued, "I know that voice...I was never afraid when I heard it, I knew you would talk to me for what seemed like hours. I didn't get nervous when I heard that voice." One of the most important aspects of critical care nursing, to me, is remembering that there is more to bringing a person back than physical health. Lungs that can oxygenate and a heart that can circulate blood are not all that make a person well.

Reflecting on some of my nursing experiences has brought "firsts" to the forefront. Early in my career, I had a memorable first Foley and IV. When I asked the patient if the IV insertion was painful, he told me, "no more painful than a lumbar puncture." In time, these practices became routine. But reminiscing also brings to mind the times when things were not routine, such as the first time we placed a patient prone in ICU because his SpO2 was so low from ARDS. One hour after the diagnosis, his condition worsened, and his life was in jeopardy. All other modalities had been attempted. Though the procedure had been carefully studied elsewhere, it had not yet been done where I was working. I remember the staff being so anxious but also so committed.

You would think they would be more committed to the procedure than the patient. But that wasn't true. It's easy to say you believe in research and evidence. Counting on those results at a crucial time is a lot more difficult. It took eight staff members, but as soon as we turned him prone, his SpO2 immediately rose. He survived. We became experts at the procedure. Not all would survive, but many more were given this one last chance.

I also recall the time we placed our first patient on the Therapeutic Hypothermia Protocol. The name has changed since, but we intentionally lowered a patient's temperature to save neurological function. Sure, the research outlined all of the benefits; we knew it well, had read it all and believed in it. We had made all of the policies and protocols based on best practices. But that was research, not someone's mother. Thankfully, this woman survived; she was discharged and went home with her family. What I think is important to have embedded in the research is this: humanity is the basis for nursing practice. Remembering and reflecting on this truth from time to time adds to our knowledge base in ways that can be incalculable, whether we are with our first or thousandth patient.

I will never forget the first time I saw CPR in action. There was a patient who was in cardiogenic shock who was admitted to the ICU. He was very sick and on a lot of medications to help maintain his blood pressure. Despite being so sick, he was awake, alert, and conversant. All of a sudden, he went into an arrhythmia on the cardiac monitor and lost consciousness. The nurses were on him almost immediately, confirmed he had no pulse, and started doing CPR. As soon as they started pumping on his chest, his face pinked up and he opened his eyes and started grunting. He was actually trying to push the nurses off of him. I felt as though I wanted them to stop. But then he went unconscious again. We shocked him once to try and get him out of ventricular fibrillation. Then we went back to doing CPR. Once again, he woke up and tried to push the nurses off of him. I was confused, yet amazed. Next they sedated him. It all happened so quickly I felt a little traumatized. I can only imagine how he felt.

This story is not about one patient or one treatment. It is about the patients who have been fortunate enough to benefit from new technology and science, such as negative-pressure wound therapy, or NPWT, unfortunate as they were for suffering from the infection in the first place. I remember watching my first application of the NWPT system and thinking it was so complicated. I could actually see this patient's ventricle moving in the hole. I hoped this would change the patient's life and wondered if the infection in his chest would really ever heal. The experts who assisted with the application boasted wound healing "in most cases." They assured us that it was not a new concept and had been around since the "Roman times." I wasn't so sure I believed that the suction used at that time actually came from soldiers' own mouths.

Although it took a long time, this patient did heal, enough to be discharged. I often wonder what that healed scar looks like. I know I won't forget what the beating of his heart looked like. Decades later, what I reflect on is this: the patients that had to heal without this device. There were so many before him who could not get this treatment, all because we had not implemented this device yet. More and more, I find myself remembering the past through these patients. We can gain so much more insight doing just that.

> *For most of human history, people died at home, within their community, or in an extraordinary circumstance such as on a battlefield. That is no longer the case. More and more, nurses and other caregivers are among the last people to see a patient before he or she passes on. It is perhaps unsurprising that for many nurses, seeing a person die for the first time is among the most memorable moments of a career. For many, there are also experiences related to death that are remarkable because of how one was able to make the end-of-life moments more peaceful or meaningful.*

He was barely alive when he came into the hospital. He had obviously not been able to do any personal hygiene in months. I heard how he was being described: homeless, unkempt, filthy. But I saw something different.

Today, we would use the words health disparity and vulnerable population. He was suffering all the same. I did what I thought would lessen his pain, alleviate his suffering. I gently bathed and shaved him. I covered him in clean sheets, warmed blankets. He died that way, about five hours after I had first met him. I felt like when he passed away, he was finally warm, clean, in a bed and he had someone with him who cared.

I have been a nurse for over twenty years. There have been many patients that I'll never forget because they helped to make me the nurse I am today. One of the most memorable patients was a man I cared for many times over the course of a three-year period. The first time I met him was after a femoral popliteal bypass surgery. He was so positive about the surgery and how it was going to improve his life. He wanted to get home to his garden, wife, and grandkids. He did well but then had to return eight months later for a revision.

The next time I cared for him, he was having some toes amputated. Once again, he was anxious to get home, but this time because his wife was sick. He was still positive and full of life. This man always had a kind word for the staff and often cheered up his roommates.

We lived in the same town, and I would occasionally run into him at the market. He always remembered me and was happy to share his progress with me. Unfortunately, his disease progressed and his wife passed away. The next time I cared for him he was very depressed. Not even his grandkids could get him out of this depression. During this hospitalization he lost his leg and this further depressed him. When he was discharged, he told the staff he was looking forward to rehabilitation and the thought of planting a garden in spring. Sadly, that was not the case. He was readmitted a few weeks later with an infection. He passed away during that admission. I remember that he always had a smile on when I entered the room.

After his passing, I sat with his daughter and we cried. I saw his daughter at the market a few months later and she thanked me again for the care and compassion I provided to her dad. During each shift that I work, I try to remember that every patient has a story to tell. They need my skill, care, and compassion to get well or die with dignity, but they also need someone to acknowledge their story.

At the time, I was just two years out of nursing school. I knew that there were many situations I had not encountered yet, death being one of them. I never expected to feel the way I did when it happened. For the first few shifts I was assigned to this patient, he was alert. Despite his diagnosis of end stage pancreatic cancer, he was talking, laughing, and so appreciative of the care he was given. His family always commented on how much he loved having me as his nurse. It was mutual. We developed that bond you can only appreciate if you are a nurse.

Then it happened. I know it was the disease, but honestly, I did not expect it. He deteriorated so fast: he was no longer speaking and barely responsive. I continued to care for him as though he was the same man. I had to talk to him and care for him. He had made me feel so important and I chose to make him feel that way now. Although his death was expected, I could not forget him. I did not sleep well for a few days. I kept thinking of how I had to cross his hands together instead of holding them. I still have a card he gave me on my bureau. It is next to my own grandmother's picture. I do not think the bond we had was simply because he was the first patient I cared for that died in my presence. I think it was he and I. That's why he is right there with my grandma's picture. I hope I gave him some happy memories and a pleasant experience despite the outcome. There have been other patients since, of course, that have passed away during my shifts. I still feel the same, and it hurts. I hope I always feel this way. They deserve it.

The patient I'll never forget is a young woman who came into my unit with a diagnosis of "vomiting." She had a three-month-old baby at home. Her husband reported that she could not stop vomiting, day and night. Several staff on my unit had suggested that "there was nothing wrong" and that maybe she was just depressed, since "that can happen" to young mothers. I learned about postpartum depression in school but I had never seen it. I knew they were wrong. Even though I had just graduated, somehow, I knew she was really sick. I saw it in her eyes. Several days later her X-ray showed an inoperable brain tumor. She never left the hospital.

I remember this patient like it was yesterday even though I cared for him more than fifteen years ago. He was admitted to the hospital with a new diagnosis of acute lymphocytic leukemia, ALL. In all, he spent three weeks in the ICU. In that time, he suffered through many complications, including pneumonia, ARDS, sepsis, and cardiogenic shock. He did not survive. We never really knew him because he was so sick when he arrived on our unit.

I remember this patient not so much for his story but because of his wife. She was one of the most caring significant others I have ever seen as a nurse. She was an advocate for her husband, a protector at all costs. In three weeks, she almost never left her husband's room. She went home just once. Every bath, treatment, and procedure was supervised by her. This woman read entire books on nursing, taken out of the library, doing her homework so she could make sure we were always following protocol. Then, after studying up on hospital policies, she made sure we followed them. As her husband's advocate, she could often be found demanding to speak to the manager of the unit or even the chief nurse of the hospital. She also told many of the nurses and therapists how inadequate they were. This quickly alienated a lot of the staff.

I honestly believe that the nurses I worked with tried very hard to care for this man in the most professional and expert way. She did not see it that way. On the day I was assigned to this patient, his wife was looking particularly exhausted. I introduced myself and she started in right away. There was a fresh list of demands: "he needs his vital signs, he needs a bath, and he needs his toupee washed, dried, and re-taped." To be clear, she wanted his toupee re-taped onto his head. I can assure you, if this man was capable, he would have ripped it off.

We had several nursing conferences on how to care for this man and his family. We had made several decisions that we all to abide by. First and foremost, his wife had to be involved in his care. None of us denied this was the right thing to do. On the day I was responsible for this man's care, I looked at his wife anew and saw fear, apprehension, and defeat. I had to fight back tears thinking about how devoted she was to the one person in her life she was about to lose. But I also thought about how she was going to need strength to endure this loss. Acting on impulse, I suggested that she not stay in the ICU that morning. She should go home and rest, have lunch, and take a shower. I promised I would care for this man as if he were mine.

She insisted she could not go.

I insisted that she could. Just before she stomped out, she asked me where the president's office was. I told her. I then gave the patient his medications, did his care, and even washed the toupee. After I put new tape inside, I made sure it was facing the right way this time. At 2 : 00 that afternoon, I saw his wife's red hair coming down the corridor. I felt badly about how I may have talked to her, or how she may have perceived it. She came so close to me I was afraid. As she got closer, I could see that she was sobbing. She embraced me and said, "You were the one that made me feel like I could leave."

After her husband passed, this woman's name would come up from time to time on the unit. Someone only had to say her first name and we all knew who we were talking about. There are not many people in the world who are known by just their first name. One of these times I remember thinking about how lucky he was. Surely, he suffered with ALL. Suffering is not a fortunate thing. It is sometimes something a nurse endures along with her/his patient. But this man was lucky enough to have someone in his life that kept his toupee on and in place no matter what. She loved him that much.

The year was 1978 and I was a recent graduate working second shift on a neurosurgical floor. My patient was a young father and husband being prepped for surgery on a brain tumor. At first our conversation was superficial as I assisted him with ADLs. Then he began to cry. I stopped what I was doing, pulled a chair up to his bedside, and reached for his hand. He held it tight. He then expressed his fears about the surgery he was going to have the following morning, wondering aloud if he would wake up the same, or wake up at all.

Then he uttered two statements through his tears that I will never forget. "I wish I took my son to one more baseball game. I wish I had told my wife I loved her one more time." Clutching his hand, I began to cry with this patient, tears rolling down my cheeks. Suddenly he let go of my hand, wiped his tears, sat up in bed and said to me, "My God woman, I'm trying to share my feelings here. Why are you crying? I'm the one going to surgery. If you can't handle this, maybe you shouldn't have become a nurse!" And there it was: my first lesson on compassion in the nursing world. He came through the surgery with no complications. I'm sure he went to many baseball games and said "I love you" many more times. As for me, I remained a handholding, tears down my cheek, kind of nurse. It's who I am. It's what we do.

Some patients never leave you. Their lives touch you in ways you never expected. My decision to move on from oncology came from caring for a young female patient diagnosed with metastatic melanoma. As if this diagnosis was not enough, this woman had recently become a mother. I will never forget this day. After her physician left the room, I came in to find her sobbing while holding her daughter. "No more treatment will help," she cried. She handed me her baby. As I held this infant and cried with my patient, my thoughts blended with hers. She would never get to raise this child. I thought that moment was frozen in my memory. Years later, I heard that her husband was tragically killed in a motor vehicle accident. I often think of their child, a daughter without parents. I wonder who is caring for her. She would be a teenager or young adult by now. This family changed my career. After this, I left oncology. There are times our connections with our patients go far beyond a single encounter.

Nurses know the methodologies to treat physical, spiritual, and emotional discomfort at the end of life. We know how to decrease fear and anxiety. We know that pastoral care affirms faith comfort. There are evidence-based strategies. We also know that comfort care is essential at the end of life. As health care providers, we are taught to relieve suffering and respect wishes. This is embedded into our practice.

The patient I won't forget had terminal melanoma, in the ICU. He was an immigrant who spoke very little English, but I understood one thing: he wanted to be married before he died. He wished for a tuxedo and to dance at his wedding. I was his nurse and I made it all happen. What I remember most was that he could barely raise his arms off the mattress due to weakness; still, he danced with his new bride. I will never forget this patient, his ceremony, or the "dance" that followed.

I think having a peaceful death is personal. I was surprised that maybe not all of my colleagues appeared to understand that. I remember all too well that some made negative comments. Some said it was unnecessary. Others reminded me to remove this man's "tuxedo."

I have been told that as a practitioner, I am too sensitive to others' misfortunes. To this day, I want to think that perhaps they did understand, but something extraneous got in the way. They did not see what I saw, which was nothing short of extraordinary. There are always needs at the beginning of life, but there are sometimes more at the end of life. Sometimes it's forgiveness, sometimes it's time for reminiscing. This patient's need was a tuxedo and a bride.

I believe this is part of the "progression of care" that nurses provide. We need to support the person behind the disease. I don't refer to patients with the name of their disease preceding them; they are human beings. I know that I am not alone in this. I also know that some disagreed with my plan to fulfill this man's wish at the end of his life. In the words of Robert Lewis: "To become what we are capable of becoming is the only end of life."

This reflection is dedicated to the memory of the patients who provided me with life-changing vision. They enriched and guided my life in ways I would have never known otherwise. My story unfolds with the thoughts of those whose misfortunes surrounded me. They granted me wisdom, restored my faith, and gave me hope for life's possibilities. My memories are filled with the patients whose life struggles and challenges still resonate with me, many years later. I begin with this reflection in the hopes that it will enlighten others about the profession of nursing. Nurses are not a gift to mankind; rather, it is those who beget suffering, difficult challenges, and loss that are the true gift to the profession of nursing.

My journey began when I was 21 years old. At such a young age I did not have much wisdom, vision, or life experience. That all changed in the years to come. The patients in this reflection (and many others) changed me and shaped my vision forever.

In my first months out of nursing school I encountered a 27-year-old patient who was partially blind, emaciated, and weak. I remember the afternoon he was admitted to my unit. He was not much older than I--how could this be? How could someone so young, like me, be so ill? After caring for him over a two-week period, I saw very little improvement in his condition. He was now headed towards dialysis for kidney failure.

Each day that I cared for him, I realized that hope is an essential part of life. Although he was blind, he never acted as if he was different. I found his strength to be amazing. He always managed to call me by my name and with a smile. One day he called me into his room to tell me he was being transferred to a different hospital called "hospice." My experience with hospice was minimal, but I knew it was a very sad journey to be traveling. This patient smiled and told me it was going to be OK, not to worry. I was heartbroken and unable to truly understand how this could be happening. I was devastated.

When I returned the next day for my assigned shift, his bed was empty. I ran to the nurse's station and inquired where he was. I was told in with a very soft voice that he had gone into failure and passed away. As tears fell from my eyes, the night nurse informed me that he'd called my name throughout the night. This was heart-wrenching to hear. I wondered what I could have done differently to enrich his life. This man's courage taught me that faith is an instrument that allows us peace. He had more life wisdom than I could ever imagine. I hold him dear to my heart, forty-one years and counting.

This patient had been admitted to my unit when she was acutely ill. I remember her frail body and lifeless posture. I understood after hearing report that she was dealing with end-stage AIDs. As I made rounds, I watched her clench her 5-year-old daughter. I remember thinking, why? How can this be? The tears falling from my eyes reminded me that love has no boundaries, nor can it be labeled. As night turned into morning, this woman held her daughter more tightly. Night after night, for ten days, I watched this woman hold her child. She passed away during this admission. To this day, I wonder about that little girl's future. This patient had taught me about the depth of a mother's love. I also learned from her that pain has no face or selection, and that no judgments should ever be made about a patient.

I sometimes felt it was always on the night shift. This patient was a new admission. My younger coworkers were struggling with seeing this 21-year-old who was actively dying. The sadness was an incredible struggle. Now as a senior nurse, they requested that I take the admission. This brought back memories of my own days as a 21-year-old nurse. I remembered the young man I had lost years ago and I took the assignment. When this patient passed away in his mother's arms that evening, I remembered the virtues my first patient had taught me. What that young mother had shown me through her strength. As I embraced the mother of this boy, I now understood the needs of my colleagues, these young, aspiring nurses.

I respected that their journey had not been quite as long as mine.

Upon completing my fortieth year in nursing, I have come to realize that this profession is enriched by those who require care, those who are learning, and those who face adversity. I have learned that patients are the ultimate teachers. They have shaped my life as a nurse, mother, nurse educator, and colleague. It was an honor to nurse these patients. My life is different because of them. I have been changed by all those whose hands I have touched. I have been honored to meet their eyes and become present based on the invitation of their hearts. With endless gratitude, I thank every patient who has touched my life and provided me with strength, wisdom, and guidance. Their lives have touched mine in ways that may have otherwise been unimaginable. Nursing has been one my life's greatest gifts.

Palliative care is specialized medical care for people with serious illness. This type of care is focused on providing relief from the symptoms and stress of a serious illness. The goal is to improve quality of life for both the patient and the family. Looking back on my experiences, I see that this a practice change that I am proud to say has evolved over the years since I first became a nurse.

I vividly remember the first time I walked into the room of a patient who had died. It was 1979. I did not expect her to look like that. The intravenous was still dripping. Her family had already gone home. I remember that her hair was black, which meant she didn't grow old enough to have gray hair. She looked frozen and alone. I realized that this was part of being a nurse. I would now have to deal with death, so I needed to keep myself together and remain calm. I still had an assignment and I did not want the other patients to know that there was a death. I recall preparing her body for the morgue, then walking with an awkward disguised stretcher through the hospital.

In another instance, I cared for a gentleman who was dying of cancer. He was fifty, strong, and muscular. He worked as a cop. He was in agony. There is no way to comfort him, physically or spiritually. The family was alone and had no support. I was young and did not know how to handle it.

In 1999, I remember my grandmother dying. She took her last breath in pain. The nurse was afraid to medicate her. I remember the nursing instructor that happened to be on the unit. She took charge and helped my grandmother, contacting the doctor and getting the medication she needed. The nurse caring for her never looked me in the eye after that. I remember holding my grandmother's hand while praying in her ear. The nursing students witnessed their instructor's intervention. I felt nurses were getting closer to figuring this out.

While caring for a patient who was a family member of a nurse on our unit, we had Led Zeppelin's "Stairway to Heaven" playing on the radio. This man died with dignity and in comfort, with his family by his side. We (nurses) were getting closer. Now I see our profession getting even closer: looking the patient and the family in the eye while talking to them about their life, accomplishments, and wishes. I see them providing palliative care. I so admire them.

Initially, I began my career in the field of pediatrics. Caring for the very young was both scary and rewarding. In the early 1970s, the case types that were cared for on the inpatient pediatric ranged from leukemia and other childhood cancers to meningitis. Skilled nurses also cared for newborns considered "border" babies. One night during a very busy shift I was assigned to the next admission to the unit. This patient happened to be a 16-year-old boy with a fever of unknown origin and abdominal pain. Right away I could see that this individual was in severe pain. No matter what medication we gave him, his pain did not go away, and I felt so helpless.

I called the Resident who was covering for the night to come up and assess the patient to be certain that there was nothing surgically wrong. The physician and I spoke to the patient and his parents and made them aware that the medication he was currently receiving was going to be administered in conjunction with another one to make him more comfortable. We would do further testing in the morning. As the night moved on my patient soon fell asleep. I checked on him often to be certain he was resting comfortably. My night shift ended but before I left for home, I went to see my patient. He was awake but comfortable. He asked if I was coming back that night to take care of him. I reassured him that I would be coming back. I could not stop thinking about him all day, wondering what tests they were performing on him and hoping he was comfortable.

That night I received my assignment. The report? This 16-year-old I had admitted the night before had a new diagnosis of liver cancer. My heart fell to the ground. I knew what this meant for him and of course his family. As time went on, I always made certain that I was his nurse, every night. Others would tell me that he would ask whether I was going to be his nurse. All the others reassured him that this is the way the assignment would be made. During one assessment, I could not believe what I saw. He was jaundice with ascites but he was sitting up in bed with a smile as I walked into the room. During the night, he would be awake on and off, complaining of discomfort. Thankfully, we were able to give him more comfort.

The most gratifying memory I have from that time of bedrest was when he pleaded with me one night to get him up to the bathroom. I felt in my heart that this needed to be done for my patient, so I asked one of my peers to assist me. We got him to the bathroom and he expressed his deepest thanks. He told us this made him feel much better and he had no pain at all. We assisted him in getting back to bed and he fell asleep without any difficulty.

The next night I came in and noticed his name was not on the assignment board. I could feel my pulse quicken and tears beginning to form. My peers quickly reassured me that the family wanted to take him home and keep him comfortable. I cried because I did not get to say goodbye.

Approximately two weeks later, I was made aware that he passed away. Some of my peers were going to his wake and I went, too. As I knelt down to pay my last respects as anyone else would do, my eyes again filled with tears. I was remembering the night I honored his simple wish to get out of bed and how happy this made him. I began to extend my sympathy to the family. As I introduced myself to his dad, someone I never had the chance to meet, he said, "so you're Donna, my son always spoke of you." He proceeded to thank me for making him comfortable. As nurses we take care of many patients, but I will always remember this young boy. This experience made me realize this is what nursing is all about and how proud I am to have made this my long-term career. Thank you for allowing me to tell my heartwarming story.

Death is an inevitable part of life. Working in healthcare reminds you of this, especially in the inpatient setting. I have been a nurse for twelve years and have worked in critical care for eleven of those years. I was an EMT for three years before that. I have seen peaceful deaths. I have seen people die in their own beds at home. I have also seen people hooked up to multiple machines and pumps in the ICU. Others have been found by family members at home on the bathroom floor. There have been people frozen solid in their cars in their driveways in winter. Others were found across a highway because of a motorcycle accident. I have seen patients die that are much younger then myself.

I often wonder how we do not become emotional disasters. I remember coming home one day, and my husband asked how my day was. I said, "It was a weird couple of days, no one died." I now explain death to my students; sometimes I think they feel I am cold and heartless because of the nonchalant way I seem to talk about death. Trust me, I am not.

I was caring for a woman in her fifties who had end-stage breast cancer. She was dying. It was the end, and she had her five daughters crowded around her at the bedside. They were all upset but had made peace with the situation. As I listened to them tell stories about her and talk about their childhood, I got to know her personality before she became ill. She was stubborn and strong and always had to have the last word. Her breathing had slowed and eventually stopped while I was in the room clearing out my IV pump for the end of my shift. I was trapped in the room behind her five daughters. But I was able to hear about what a wonderful mother she was. They thanked her for everything she had done for them, and they all said goodbye. I was silently weeping, listening to them talk to her. There was a moment of silence after they all got finished talking and she took one more breath. All five girls burst out laughing and looked at me and said, "See! Always has the last word!" I remember thinking about how sad it was, but how people can still laugh at the end when the most horrible things are happening around them.

I took care of a woman who was in her eighties and dying from a small bowel obstruction. She was not a surgical candidate due to her multiple comorbidities. This woman had a nasogastric (NG) tube to suction. She was delirious. At times I am thankful for delirium; it may mean that people are not aware of what is happening to them.

When I walked into the room, she was smiling from ear to ear and reaching around in the air like she was trying to catch something. I asked her how she was feeling and if she was having any pain. She said, "No, but I am having trouble, can you help me?" I noticed she was not looking at me at all, but I asked what she needed help with. She replied, "There is too much cotton candy! I can't get it all in the bag!" She died about eight hours later; she went to sleep and drifted away. I remember thinking that cotton candy may not be a bad hallucination at the end of life.

Working in a cardiac ICU, I see a lot of patients who are very sick and need cardiac surgery. Severe alcohol and IV drug use can lead to severe heart failure as well as septic endocarditis, a blood infection that settles on the valves of the heart and eats away at them. Often these patients need cardiac surgery to replace valves and, in some cases, parts of their aorta. I work with the adult population because I could not care for children who are seriously ill. Patients in their late teens, barely adults, are difficult for me as well. I once took care of a 19-year-old male patient who was admitted with septic endocarditis from IV drug use with an abscess around his aortic valve. He had undergone cardiac surgery just a year and a half earlier to have his aortic valve, and part of his ascending aorta replaced because of another episode of endocarditis. The surgeons at the time told him that they could fix him, but he would have a new valve and so much graft material inside his aorta that if he ever did IV drugs again and got re-infected, there was nothing they could do, and he would not be a surgical candidate. He agreed and went into rehab after he was discharged home post-surgery.

Within two months he had relapsed and started doing IV drugs again. He'd become reinfected with bacteria, but this time attached to the graft material that was lining his aorta. There was no cure. I sat in as the surgeon came in to speak with him. He asked him what happened. The patient said, "You know, I made a mistake. I remember what you said, but I figured you were just saying that to scare me to try and get me on the right path." The surgeon responded, "I did say that to scare you, but not to put you on the right path, to save your life. You didn't take me seriously, and that was a mistake. I can't operate on you again; there is nothing I can do. We will give you antibiotics to try and treat the infection, but that is just to make you feel better, it is not going to help. You have a new pathway in the form of an abscess around the valve I replaced that will eventually let go. We don't know when it is going to happen, but it will. I am sorry to see you back here. Let me know if there is anything, I can do to help make you more comfortable." The patient didn't say anything, and the surgeon left.

This is the part where the nurses step in. We catch the questions the patient didn't think to ask or was afraid to ask while the surgeon was there. I stayed behind to make sure the patient and his girlfriend understood what was said. She said, "what a jerk," and asked for a new doctor. She was very young and the only support system he had. We learned he had distanced himself from his family and wouldn't tell us who they were or where they were. I asked him what he thought about what the surgeon said. He just looked at me for a minute and asked me if he was kidding. I said no, this is not a joke. There is nothing funny about it. I asked him if there were any family members that he would like me to contact and offered him support services as well. He declined. I stayed with him.

He finally looked at me and said, "So I am really going to die? I don't understand. I don't feel that sick...is this something that I can just stay on antibiotics for a few years or something?" I told him no and that he won't be able to leave the hospital. His girlfriend began to scream at me, she asked me to leave the room. I gave them time to process before I went back in. He said that he still refused to believe it. He was too young, he was strong, and he would be fine.

The next morning, very early, one of my colleagues was seen running out of his room. "He doesn't look good. He is having chest pain." Diaphoretic and gray, he kept saying, "something's not right, help me." Patients are usually right about this. His arterial blood pressure dropped. His ECG waveform changed and eventually flattened out. He went from sitting up in bed to laying back. He was gone. Alone, except for me. No family. I just watched someone's son die and they didn't even know. In the aftermath, it was thought that the abscess ruptured, or he bled.

Dealing with this is not something that you can be taught. Professors and other nurses can talk to you about what to expect as a nurse, but you really don't understand until you live it. There are times you feel that you may be pushed to your limit of suffering, when you experience too many deaths. Compassion Fatigue is what they call it now. It's both physical and emotional. I can see how it happens. I don't think I am "there" yet. At the point where I can't see it anymore. I'm keeping watch on it, though. I have a comfort with death at this point, which in itself makes me uncomfortable.

I had not seen death before this. I was a volunteer working towards becoming an EMT. I had no intention of working on an ambulance or being a nurse for that matter, but here I was working on a student-run ambulance. This is what happens when your best friend wants to do something, but "not alone." Within my third shift as a volunteer, it happened. The call. We heard: "Unresponsive male, outside one of the dorm buildings." The seasoned EMT responded differently than I: rolling his eyes, "great, welcome to college ambulance runs, your first of many. Drinking." My friend and I had not even mastered taking a blood pressure yet.

I saw a young man on the ground, a police officer hunched over him. It was dark, it was after midnight, my eyes trying to adjust. I remember thinking, "What is he doing?"

It was CPR. My stomach clenched as I approached the lifeless college student. I heard him on the radio calling for advanced life support mutual aid from the neighboring town. He pointed to me. "Stand there and hold his neck straight. Don't move." I watched as a team continued CPR, IVs, medications, intubated, all concurrently asking "what happened?" I stood and held his bloody head. I remember how pale he was and how weird his stomach looked bobbing up and down as he was getting CPR. He was so limp.

It was a dorm party. He had fallen off a third-floor balcony. He was not even a student at this university; he was visiting from out of state. My friend and I had actually been to the same dorm about an hour earlier. We'd taken a girl into the hospital who was having back pain.

He didn't live. This was almost the end of my career. I had doubts this would be the career for me.

It is hard to believe that more than thirty-five years have passed since I graduated with a baccalaureate degree in nursing. So many practice changes have occurred in this time; however, the profession of nursing remains an art and a science. When writing this story, one cannot help but review the American Nurses Association definition: "nursing is the protection, promotion, and optimization of health and abilities, prevention of illness and injury, alleviation of suffering through the diagnosis and treatment of human response, and advocacy in the care of individuals, families, communities, and populations." The patient I can't forget was a woman diagnosed with parotid cancer. She received her chemotherapy regimen each month as an inpatient on a surgical unit with primary nursing at its best. As a professional nurse with less than two years of experience, I provided holistic and compassionate care. I was new to the practice of nursing. It was hard knowing that this disease was aggressive, but each interaction was simple because this patient was optimistic. She lived life to the fullest. Despite being nauseous and sick from the chemotherapy she was always grateful for the care and compassion provided her. Knowledge of the disease process, the medications administered, and the rationale for her care, were all important. However, the most rewarding part of caring for her came when I was sitting eye level, serving as an intentional presence providing comfort and discussing her plan of care, her family, and special events in her life. She taught me to be more compassionate than I already was.

Clinical expertise is vitally important, but so are the human connections that nurses make inside and outside of the hospital.

My patient suffered complications from a gastric bypass surgery that nearly took her life. Caring for her each day was challenging, but she never gave up. Smiles and positivity were important to her care. This patient's nurses and other healthcare team members became her family. She required long dressing changes, multiple antibiotics, total parenteral nutrition, and help moving from bed to chair with a lift. This woman had a complex treatment plan, but she received excellent care and was discharged home one year later. She was able to walk and care for herself independently. The care team held a going home party. This patient taught me to be more resilient and to never, ever give up.

Approximately twelve years later, I was fortunate to have a CNO who can be described as a thought leader. She was a role model: a source of inspiration who exhibited a passion for excellence. She identified the organization's culture that valued nursing and she initiated the Magnet® journey. I earned a master's degree in nursing administration, so I worked with her CNO and the team and three years later the hospital was designated Magnet® Recognition for nursing excellence and 4 years later re-designated.

The evolution of Magnet® began as a research study to identify the characteristics of a work environment that retains and recruits the best nurses. This work and the Magnet® Recognition Program clearly identifies the value of nursing, the importance of a work environment that supports excellence in nursing and has elevated nursing practice in a positive way. Practice changes based on evidence and the expansion of nursing research activities places nurses at an equal partnership with physicians and other medical professionals. For more than twenty years, my work in nursing has been linked to Magnet® with pride.

Magnet® Recognition is really about the patients, families, communities, and populations; it is the quality of care nurses provide with the entire team and within a supportive environment.

To me, nursing means being kind, innovative, compassionate, and trustworthy; it also means being aware of best practices and translating new knowledge into practice through critical thinking.

Looking back on my career, I see how patients from my past shaped me as a nurse and a person. These experiences made me realize that being a nurse was the right profession. Patients would look to me to protect, promote, and optimize their health and abilities. Some needed me to alleviate suffering and advocate for the best care possible, but I also looked to them as individuals who were courageous and inspiring.

Every nurse has cared for patients they will never forget. Many patients have me as a person. Always being a hard-working individual, it was the experiences of being part of these patients' lives that showed me that life is precious and that every day is one to cherish.

Writing this story at a time when I am much older brings a greater awareness that life is not forever and it is important to enjoy every moment. Nurses make a difference as advocates in the care of patients and families and I'm grateful to have chosen this profession and to have had these special moments. These experiences taught me that values are important in life and to the profession. People often say "Life is a journey, not a destination." Mostly, though, it means being true to oneself by encouraging everyone to always strive for excellence. Because patients deserve the highest quality care.

***Nurses who are used to thinking
of friends, colleagues, or others in their
lives in one way sometimes see that
relationship transformed into a bond forged in caregiving.***

I recently retired from my position as a nurse at a health services and women's clinic. In that role, I assisted physicians and nurse practitioners in caring for many wonderful and interesting students, some of whom were studying nursing at the college. Some students I would see often over their four years and their faces and stories became familiar to me. Educating these young women was a great opportunity and true joy.

I recently saw some of these same women again when I was hospitalized for an emergency surgery, resulting in a three-week stay. Three of my nurses on the floor where I was treated had been nursing students at the institution where I worked at the clinic. All three remembered me and commented on the kindness of the staff at the clinic. They talked about the care and compassion shown to them, the treatment and education they received, and what it meant to be able feel better and return to their studies.

What I needed to share is that I received the same, not only from these three nurses, but everyone on the staff. It's different to be on the other side, to be vulnerable, fearful, and not knowing. It did not matter that I had forty years of experience in nursing. I was scared. But I was cared for, educated, treated, and reassured. In the end, I was able to return to my blessed life. As one of these graduates put it, "You took wonderful care of me, now it's my turn to care for you."

He wasn't assigned to me, at least not in the usual nurse-patient sense. This patient was a best friend. We stood up for each other at our weddings. We traveled together, we dreamed together. He visited me on my days off. There is one visit I can't forget. It was the visit that changed our friendship, the one where I became his nurse. I was folding laundry that day he knocked on the door.

Usually, he came bearing iced tea, a small gift for me. That day, he didn't; that day, I saw a pale, worried friend. He immediately jumped into the conversation. That part wasn't unusual. It was when he asked me to look at his abdomen that everything changed. From the nipple line to the hips, he was completely ecchymotic, his body severely discolored. He asked, "What do you think?" I knew immediately that he was dying. I think he knew, too.

About thirteen months later he was buried, after a battery of blood transfusions, tests, infusions, and injections. Though aplastic anemia is curable in some, it was not in my friend. During those thirteen months, he often looked to me for answers. But his questions were not obvious. The questions were hidden, woven into general conversations that you may have had at any other time in life. That was his way of making this easier for me. Perhaps he was even more of a friend than I'll ever imagine. He never asked me if I thought he was going to die. I don't think he needed to. I was his friend for many years and his nurse for only thirteen months. I hope he thinks I did my best.

I worked at a community hospital in the ICU when I was a relatively new nurse, and I loved my job. Working with and caring for people in the community was always something that I enjoyed. There was often a personal connection between staff and patients and because of that, there was a different kind of comfort and trust between staff, patients, and families. There were also times that the connections hit a little bit too close to home.

I was 30 years old in 2009 when I cared for a patient I will never forget. He was 87 years old and had been admitted to the hospital for a colostomy reversal which was initially placed when he was undergoing radiation therapy for rectal cancer. He had a successful resection of the tumor and completed radiation treatment, but he did not want to live out the rest of his life with the colostomy. He came into the hospital in decent health and good spirits without a lot of major comorbidities. He had the colostomy reversal procedure done and was admitted to the med /surg floor postoperatively. He had a fairly unremarkable immediate post-operation course. He woke up and came out of anesthesia without any confusion or delirium and had adequate pain management.

A few days after his procedure, he developed a low-grade fever, got some Tylenol, and settled in for the night. The nurses went into his room to assess him in the middle of the night and found him nearly unresponsive, and they called a rapid response, which was when the ICU team got involved. He was in septic shock. He was intubated for oxygenation and airway protection. He was given fluid resuscitation and required a central line placement to receive vasopressors to support his blood pressure. Attempts were made to call family early in the morning after he was transferred to the ICU; however, they were unable to reach the primary next of kin.

They called the second number, and there was no answer, so they called back the primary number and left a message with the patient's daughter to please call back as soon as possible. Septic shock in an 89-year-old. The outcome is guarded. I was scheduled to work the night shift that first night after he was transferred to the ICU. I saw a missed phone call from work. I called them back figuring they were busy and wanted me to work the day shift instead of the night or wanted me to come in early. One of my co-workers answered the phone, and I asked her if anyone had called me. She asked around, said no one called me, but they were very busy at work so if I wanted to come in early, she was sure no one would say no. I told her I would check back around lunchtime to see how things were going. My mom called me a little bit later in the morning, and she sounded upset. "Can you come to the hospital? Your grandfather got pretty sick last night with an infection, and he got transferred to the ICU. I am on my way in to see him now." The phone call I had missed that morning was the covering hospitalist calling me because my mom hadn't answered the phone when they called overnight. They didn't leave a message.

My grandfather was born and raised in a small village. He moved later on to become a prospector in Alaska. He was a pilot in WWII, had a distinguished career as a First Lieutenant, flew a P 51 Mustang, over 50 missions. For his military service, he received the Air Medal with Four Oak Leaf Clusters and the Distinguished Flying Cross. He met my grandmother during the war, they were married for 60 years. He became a Pharmacist. He opened up his own pharmacy when my mother was born. He volunteered; his passion was providing medicine and pharmaceutical services for the poor and underserved populations in the islands. He was the only grandparent that I got to know as an adult. Then he was diagnosed with rectal cancer.

My mother and I took turns taking him to the hospital for diagnostic testing, surgical procedures, and radiation treatments. We helped him apply medications to rectal radiation burns and watched him grow weak and tired, as he was in constant pain. The nurse in me was fine with giving him personal care; the granddaughter in me was not. Granddaughters aren't supposed to give personal care to a war hero. He died a month after the reversal of his colostomy. I watched him intubated, extubated and re-intubated several times. His vocal chords were damaged because of the breathing tube, and he was never able to speak again.

He was so weak, his body was so swollen, he couldn't move his arms enough to write.

Enteral feedings, frequently suctioned. It was now his life. For the three weeks he was in ICU, my role was confusing. I helped turn him, and bathe him, and clean him, and suction his airway. I felt guilty being there and taking care of other patients.

I know he could see me sitting out at the nurse's station charting and always wondered what he was thinking. Did he wish I was in his room more, or less? Did he enjoy just watching me work and care for others? Not many family members get that inside view of what you do when you work in the nursing profession. He had been intubated "too long." "Time for a tracheostomy." The war hero had suffered; maybe it was enough. In the end, his breathing tube was removed, and he was breathing on his own, though he had a very weak cough and still had to be suctioned frequently, which he hated. He was finally stable enough to be transferred out of the ICU to the medical floor.

The phone call I got this time was from my nurse manager. I was coming in to work that night, so I thought the phone call might be work-related. "Liz, I just wanted to let you know that they are transferring your grandfather out of the ICU to the floor." Time for conversations about code status. Throughout all of this debilitating illness he had, he was mentally always entirely cognizant. We approached the topic with him and the Physician. He asked my grandfather if his heart stopped or he had trouble breathing if he wanted to have CPR done and have a breathing tube placed back in. He looked at my mother, who had been with him every moment, every step of the way, late nights, early mornings, making sure there was someone with him as much as possible.

My mother laughed and said, "Don't do this for me! What do YOU want!" He shook his head no, we smiled and cried at the same time, and changed his code status to a DNR /DNI.

He died two days later. He remained the independent man he always was. He was alone, and we think that was alright for him. But not for us. The message came but we were too late. I knew it as soon as I looked into his room. He was peaceful. Positioned perfectly, oxygen still on, his hand neatly folded. Family pictures were placed on the bedside table. It was just how a family would want to see the room of a loved one being taken care of. I'm not sure the staff knew, but I knew. I let my mom know before she went in. I let the staff know, after they asked if there was something I needed. I tactfully said, "Well, we just came in to visit my grandfather and found him dead, so I just wanted to make sure someone knows. We will be in the room."

It sounds very bitter on paper, but I promise, it was not said with any spite or negativity. Despite us and staff being with him almost constantly, he waited until no one was there, not even his nurse, to die.

The biggest regret I have is that at some point, my grandfather asked for a strawberry milkshake, but couldn't have it because he couldn't swallow. I wish I could have gotten him one. For months after that driving back and forth over the bridge between my house and the hospital where I worked, each time I drove over the bridge when it was dark, one street light would flicker on as I drove by. It wasn't always the same one, but I always noticed one. For some reason, whenever this happened, I would think of my grandfather. This experience that I had with him in the hospital has forever impacted the way that I interact with my patients and their family members who are critically ill and in end of life situations.

I am now a Nurse Practitioner and have worked with some of the sickest people, with the majority of my time spent in large tertiary care centers, cardiothoracic surgical ICU, heart and lung transplants, valvular repairs, CABG. I now initiate and continue to have these hard end-of- life discussions with patients and family members. My goal is to provide to them the support, information, and comfort just like I received when my loved one was this ill.

In the end, nursing is about relationships. After all of the medications are disbursed, the procedures are completed, the paperwork is done, and EMR fields filled in, many nurses are still not "done" with those they care for. In fact, going above and beyond to make "life worth living," as one contributor put it, is often a daily practice.

I used to work nights at a facility with a unit for long-term disabled adults. These patients could not physically care for themselves; at times they could not even perform ADLs and definitely not their IADLs. But it is not always the physical disability that challenges us to care for those assigned to us. Though they are suffering from chronic conditions, often, in patients like the one I will describe, they are not aware of it.

Disabilities are so often psychological or psychiatric in long term care. This can make our role so much more challenging, but somehow exciting.

Though it has been years, I still often think of this one patient. I no longer work on his unit, but I wonder who he calls at 8 : 00 p.m. or who he "tells" now. This man was my patient every night from 11 a.m. - 7 p.m. That was my assignment and my shift, but that was not his assignment. He needed me to know when he went to the bathroom, even if I wasn't there. "Be sure to tell her; I know she is not here to see it," he would warn the other nurses.

He couldn't go to bed without calling me. At 8 : 00 p.m. every night, he would ask the other nurses to call me before he went bed. They were sure that without this phone call, he would not have gone to bed. So, I would faithfully answer the phone, even on my nights off. I would tell him every day that it was a good time to lay down. I could not imagine not answering the phone.

My responsibilities as a nurse reached out a little farther than the eight hour shift I was paid for, but for this patient, it made all the difference. Success in nursing is relative. I think it is especially rewarding to be successful as a nurse in long-term care. For people unable to live outside of an institution, it is our role to make that life worth living.

I was a student nurse when a young patient was admitted to the Emergency Department with the diagnosis of GSW, a gunshot wound. Someone called out: "Compressions in progress!" Then he arrived. I could not help but think: he is perfect. He is a perfect 16-year-old, on the outside. I will never forget how I found out he was perfect on the inside, too. I watched and looked as they performed a resuscitative thoracotomy. His entire chest opened up, like a clamshell. There it was, a perfect pericardium, a perfect heart, perfect lungs. A perfect face, a beautiful child. I will never forget him.

You usually have to work the night shift as a new graduate. I was caring for an older gentleman in a Step-Down Cardiac unit. One night I found this man wide awake at 3:00 am. He told me he couldn't sleep. The unit was the "Q" word, the one you never say, (quiet) that night. I decided to spend time with him. I did my charting next to him, chatted for quite a long time. I'll never forget how proud he was when he told me he knew Rodney Dangerfield. I remember how much he looked like he truly enjoyed my company. Sometimes when you separate the tasks from the job, just for a short time, you're amazed at the moments of caring that happen.

This happened more than twenty years ago, but if I close my eyes, I can still hear it. I describe it as the sound you hear when water/condensation builds up in the corrugated tubing attached to the humidifier of oxygen. They used to call it "rain-out." It gurgles, pops, it will spit at you if you disconnect it wrong. The noise is louder than you would think. The noise is unmistakable, almost.

I was 23 years old this time when I heard it. It wasn't the corrugated tubing, but I thought it was. It was in the pediatric ICU, I heard it immediately when the automatic doors opened. I asked the RN why someone couldn't empty that tubing. "It isn't water in a tubing. It's a child. It's breathing. It's end of life." I immediately thought there must be a solution, something I could do. It was then I decided that there must always be a solution to alleviate symptoms, no matter what they are. There may not be chemotherapy, biotherapy, or radiation. But there's solutions to symptoms if you look hard enough. I now care for children who need palliative care. My mission is to always find the solution to symptoms for these children. My thoughts often go back to that noise I thought was the corrugated tubing. It's been more than 20 years and I can still hear it. I never even knew this child's name, gender or age, but I often wonder what this child's parents remember hearing.

I was working in the emergency department as a new graduate nurse, with less than a year of experience. There was a specific patient that I remember and have thought about more than any other. She was in her early fifties and complaining of chest pain. The CT scan showed a ruptured aortic dissection. This is life-threatening and the plan was to transfer her for quaternary care. While all this was happening, she requested to see her three teenage sons. The patient told me she wanted to tell her boys of her uncertain situation. She knew that she didn't have much time and all she could think was that this could be her last possible moments with them. When her sons arrived, she wanted to impart a few life observations to make them better men. She pleaded with them to be good to other people, to remember the good times the family had shared, to always be gentlemen and open doors for women, not to forget their wives' birthdays or anniversaries, do well in school. Above all, never forget how much that she loved them. This was very emotional for me, being the mother of young boys also. This was the first time I had shed tears for one of my patients. I do not know what happened to her after she was transferred. As I write this story, I can't help but shed more tears.

Chapter Four

Collegiality & Practice

Jeannine Borozny, Leiah Gallagher, Donna Horrocks,
Rachel Jones, Rebecca Jones, Ellen O'Rourke,
Angela Quarters, Deb Quirk,
Rosemary Walker, Ginny Wilcox

"Alone we can do so little, together we can do so much."

Helen Keller

Anyone who works in the medical profession will tell you that some of what happens at work must stay at work. There are legal reasons for this, of course. Protecting a patient's privacy is paramount in nursing, and it is a cornerstone of modern professionalism. Yet there are also profound emotional experiences at work that often stay compartmentalized. The impulse to do this is not so much legal or ethical but emotional. Trying days and draining caregiving experiences can end up staying at work—and with colleagues—because they are too difficult to also deal with at home.

The highs and lows of nursing form a special bond between colleagues. Nurses do not merely work somewhere. When they show up, they perform complex intellectual and interpersonal processes in environments that really are unlike any other. Nurses often do their jobs in busy places—hospitals, clinics, and other settings that are filled with other professionals. They are never truly working alone. Day or night, they are surrounded by colleagues, including fellow nurses, physicians, patients, families, and so on. But some of the most important people in a nurse's life are those who have walked the same, or a similar path. In this densely packed ecosystem, nurses have a particular relationship with one another that defies easy categorization. Through night shifts, blizzards, and other extraordinary times, nurses come to understand one another.

The bonds that form among nurses at and around the bedside are without parallel. They also extend beyond work. During some of the most trying times in an individual's life, nurses can support one another in ways that others might find incomprehensible. As one contributor explained, "they know you." Particularly when a colleague is ill, the shared connection between nurses spills over into life, going beyond the long shifts they shared at their job. Nursing can truly be the source of lifelong friendships that bring empowerment and sustenance.

These stories clearly show that nurses can serve as mentors, lifting one another up. They can push each other through difficult times and to new heights as professionals. Yet nurses can also be responsible for deeply damaging work environments, and for causing lateral violence and other difficulties. All of this must be understood within the context of the intensity of the bond that nurses share; like any relationship, it is not entirely positive or negative. From novice to retired expert, nurses experience closeness and by extension, friction. In examining their own relationships with colleagues through the years, these contributors put the range of emotions that comes with being a fellow nurse into sharper view.

In these stories, nurses express their profound gratitude for the mutual understanding they have shared with colleagues in and out of work through the years.

I think that your colleagues in nursing are like no other colleagues. They are your lifeline, they are your spirit, they are bound up with you. They understand what others do not. They know that there are many patients that you will care for that will never recover, whether from alcoholism, substance abuse, or cancer. They also know how close we all are to being there ourselves, because any one of these can happen to us, and it has. That's why you don't judge—you can't. We don't judge the 18-year-old who took four bottles of Tylenol and went to bed. We don't judge the mother who checked on her fifteen hours later, too late for her to recover. We can't judge ourselves when, after many doses of acetylcysteine solution this beautiful 18-year-old high school senior has liver failure. Many of your colleagues have 18-year-olds at home. You don't say a word, but you all leave this shift together, walking out in a group with "the look." We all know the look, it is weighed down with the unasked question of why. All we can do now is go home a little faster to see your own 18-year-old.

When I was faced with the devastating diagnosis of breast cancer, my colleagues stood by me. I worked in Pediatrics at the time, my love. During surgical treatment, chemotherapy and radiation, my colleagues took me to appointments. They insisted on having tea every week; they insisted I attend. They worked extra shifts when my job was threatened. I was out of work for nine months. My nurse manager called every week. They saved me in more ways that I can describe. This was many years ago, but I will never forget what they did for me.

I had been a nurse for a long time. I had watched my own children being born (when I wasn't screaming). But when my daughter was about to give birth it was different. The happy couple asked me to be present at the birth. I, of course, did research. Would this be good for their family? I talked to my colleagues in obstetrics and they gave me sources of research to read. I learned the most important thing was not to interfere in their new family. The day finally came, and when my first grandson was born, I could not have been happier. He was perfect.

It's what happened just before he was born that was incredible. There were things about that birth that no one else even noticed, except me. The parents never knew how my daughter's nurse managed to monitor the heart rate of two people. Nor did they know how the nursing team managed the oxygen levels of my daughter, my new grandson and, the status of my son-in-law, who looked like a sheet of paper, absolutely drenched in sweat, almost not vertical.

The nurses managed to do all of these things seamlessly, including something I will never forget as long as I live. The new parents never noticed that the nurse asked me if I wanted to touch my grandchild before he was born. My grandson is now 10 years old, and every time I see him, I remind him I was the first person in the whole world to touch him. I couldn't love him more. For all of my OB nurse colleagues, you knew I would feel this way. You inspire me.

It's strange, but there are some things that happen while you are a nurse that you just can't explain at home. I still think about this one particular 85-year-old patient who was brought from an emergency room after receiving tPA for an ischemic stroke. As I was walking alongside the stretcher, she held her husband's hand the whole way. The next part was routine as I settled her into the room in intensive care. I took her blood pressure and heart rate, and then I looked at her pupils, asked her to grasp my hands and last, to stick her tongue out. Her husband of sixty years interjected: "she is really good at that." After they laugh, he kissed her, told her he loves her, and that he "will always love her."

She says she loves him back. I can't explain to anyone, even my husband, how I felt about what happened next. As I left the room to get a computer to chart this admission, I reached the threshold, and heard him scream. He cried out, "She's gone!" She had died of an intracerebral hemorrhage. Privacy is only one reason why I can't talk to my husband about this. It's because he doesn't look at the veins. Instead, I talk to my colleagues, because they do look, and they understand. If I could not do that, I could not have returned the next day or the day after that. Turning to a colleague, feeling the swelling in my throat, I said, "He was going to love her forever." All she had to say was "he did," but it was enough.

My colleagues knew things. Sometimes they know more than anyone else in your life about you, because they know how much you appreciate life, how you feel about death, how much you don't want to see suffering, and how hard you will work to have your patient not be in pain. They knew about me expecting my last child before I did; I swore it could not be the reason I was so sick. They also knew how I wanted to be told that my own mother, who had been admitted to intensive care, no longer had a rhythm on the monitor.

Your colleagues are not your friends and they are not your family. They are somewhere in between, in there with you as a nurse. They know you. They come to your father's funeral and stand in a perfect row, in uniform. They know you. They do exactly the right things when a multiple trauma puts you in a wheelchair for seven months. They know you, so they send you a card every day for seven months. You know them, too. You know when they feel they fall short of perfect, just like you do sometimes. You know when to gather and unify when one of you needs it. There is not much discussion, you just do it. It's like family, but not, like best friends, but not. They just know you.

I will never forget the day everyone was so worried about a colleague. Someone noted that she "just wasn't herself today." Another nurse observed, "or yesterday." I was with her during a patient admission from the emergency room to the intensive care unit. Together, we transferred the patient onto the bed from the stretcher. Then she stared at me, crying. She was holding a pulse oximeter in her hand. After many years of clinical practice, she had no idea what to do with it. I knew instantly. I hoped it was not true, but I knew. Our colleague died a few months later of cancer. I think just about every nurse in our hospital drove her at least once to therapy, the market, or radiation in those few months. I know for certain that everyone that was not on duty stood in line at the funeral.

What does it mean to be successful as a nurse and as a colleague? These reflections offer important insights into the value of appreciating one another's gifts and contributions.

After 41 years of a bedside nursing career, I have had my heart open and seen humanity shine. Along my path, I have seen moments of humor, dedication, and wonder. I have seen colleagues cheer each other on, learn from one another, and offer moral support. But there's one that did all of this, and more, and made a difference in my life: Joanie. She has a presence like no other. She affectionately gave everyone a nickname, making them feel like her special friend. Everyone wanted to be her friend, and her colleague. From environmental services to the radiology department, every staff member knew her. And she knew them.

Knowing isn't always respecting, but in Joanie's case, it was. And it was mutual. Joanie wasn't just the caregiver who gave you a nickname, however. She was the one all of us would ask for when we were sick. She managed her patients. She showed everyone that was new the ways to treat people. She shared. We often thought she was the most efficient person we ever worked with. Some of us thought it was her cart. One thing you needed to know about that cart: do not touch it. Ever. It was why she was efficient. She stocked it at the beginning of the shift. It had everything you needed to care of the patient.

Joanie nicknamed herself "Meme." Patients asked if Meme was working. Staff asked if Meme was working. They knew it would be a good night if Meme was on. Joanie brought her skills to several different roles in her career. Not just the cart skills, but her skills of making all who came in contact feel important. Meme named me "Rosebud" a long time ago. It was close to my name, but so much more endearing.

Success can be seen in many forms, including the way you live and the way you treat others. Joanie has recently had serious illness herself. Despite this, she continues to shine. She continues to make everyone around her feel special. It's not just the new name she will give you, it's her. Thank you, my friend, my colleague, Meme.

There are the patients who are so critically ill that almost no one expects them to survive. But with a team of people from various disciplines who are diligent and relentless in their efforts to save this patient, the patient survives and comes back to visit when they are well. That is the ultimate in happiness. The list could go on and on. To me, nursing means learning and research and teamwork and the sacred opportunity to connect with the patients and their families when they are most vulnerable.

There are also endless opportunities available to nurses. There are nursing specialties such as emergency nursing, critical care nursing, surgical nursing, pediatric nursing, and obstetrical nursing. There are roles for staff nurses, managers, directors, chief nursing officers and nurse practitioners. The road is not always easy; there are certainly challenges along the way. But I can tell you that I would choose the same career today as I chose many years ago. The support and camaraderie I have found in nursing is invaluable to me and I am fortunate to have a career that I love.

For me, personally, satisfaction in my career has always come from helping others. I found this to be especially true at the end of my career, in an inner-city hospital, with a patient population I found to be the most satisfying to care for. The nurses I worked with never called their patients "frequent flyers." They embodied compassionate care beyond what I saw at any other time in my career. I once observed a nurse running from the emergency room with a wheelchair and blankets to pick up a patient off of the sidewalk. He had either walked out of the emergency room or just landed on the sidewalk. He was a person who lived in the neighborhood. I watched as she put her arm around him, wrapped him in a blanket, and asked him if he was cold. Then she asked him what happened. She looked directly at him to say, "you always know where to land, and you know we'll care about you. Let us help you."

Nurses work together in a broader clinical context; as previously noted, they are also in a larger work system. In relation to other professionals, how nurses relate to doctors has changed significantly through the years. Notably, nurses also have shifting relationships with other personnel, including staff secretaries.

I could write many pages about the delicate relationship between nurses and doctors. To begin with, I will never understand why a chart had to be thrown at me. The order the physician wrote said to hold the Heparin for aPT T>50 seconds, so I held it, and I called him. The patient's aPT T was 50. But even as the chart was flying by my head, I remember thinking the doctor really does want what is best for this patient with a deep vein thrombosis (DVT). From my first week after graduation when this physician threw the chart at me, to the many times I have been asked my opinion for the best care for the patient, I am grateful to know this relationship. I will forever admire the physicians I have worked with during my career.

Physicians have always been part of our landscape, but relationships between physicians and nurses are very different now. In the 1970s, nurses at the nurses' station got up from their chairs when the physicians needed to sit down. My years working in intensive care have showed me the best that physicians have to offer. I have admired the many physicians who were not only there for the patient but equally for their loved ones. Physicians are as human as the rest of us. It was not easier for them simply because they were more educated.

I was the RN. She was working as a secretary on the same unit. I would remember how she would always say, "I don't want to be like you." But eventually she enrolled in nursing school, graduated and began her career in the same hospital as I was in. Sometimes I would visit her when I was leaving for the day and she had just begun her shift. One day I stood outside a patient's room and I could hear her as she cared for a patient. I was amazed. Her compassion, her skill, as I waited, I would hear her caring for her patient. She never knew I was there. I began to think, she has made me so proud, so happy. But I think more important was how much she loved her new role. It made me think of something she had said about not wanting to be like me. She must have known she was just like me. We both found our love.

Nurses do not work traditional business hours. They spend long nights, weekends, and holidays at work with one another. The particular stresses of working at night put a strain on the body and mind that can be especially difficult to cope with. As these stories suggest, many a friendship has been formed with eyes half-closed.

Working nights forms a unique camaraderie. You completely understand the extreme fatigue no matter how many hours you sleep. Your whole life is based on "how many hours did you get?" I recall eating salsa and guacamole at 4 : 00 a.m. and the ten-minute car naps that temporarily felt like hours of sleep. Working at night means combating the body's natural rest period while trying to remain alert and high functioning. It doesn't matter whether night nurses get enough sleep during the daytime. All the sleep in the world does not help.

The circadian misalignment is real, but it is also so much more than that. When I was working nights, I was also caring for my parents. For some reason my mom would "worry" about me and have to "test" the bell I gave her to call me if there was an emergency. She tested it about six times during the only hour of sleep I was going to get until after dinnertime.

It's really the "best shift for everyone," except the one who is working it. When your children are young and you work 11 p.m. – 7 a.m., you try to find a few minutes for sleep during the day. Sometimes you're in luck, most times you're not. One of the most annoying things about that quick sleep you may get is when (after one hour) everyone asks you how your "nap" was. You think to yourself: this was not a nap. It's all the sleep I've had in thirty-six hours.

Particularly when you work nights and have young children, strange things happen. I heard of one of my colleagues waking up to at least fifty marbles in her hair, one in each curl. Another colleague woke up to find her two boys out in the street giving each person going by a check from her checkbook. I dozed off one day after a twelve-hour night shift and woke up to find my in-laws sitting next to me; despite the drool, there I was, in my nightgown, apparently ready to receive visitors. My children had graciously let them in.

The holidays are different for a night person. You have to work "the night before" or "the night of." That's just the way it is. So, in every holiday picture your eyes are closed or half closed. Food during the holidays takes on a whole different meaning, too. The buffet you and your colleagues eat at 3: 00 a.m. sounds good at the time but it does not mix well with the turkey you need to prepare and get into the oven when you get home. Then there is the dreaded recycled buffet, the food that is put out for the next round of colleagues. Most nurses would agree, though, that even if life is harder, night colleagues are the best.

When I graduated from nursing school, I had to take a self-assessment to determine if I was a morning person or a night person. I remember thinking this was futile since I was going to have to work overnights either way. The test related your sleeping habits to birds. I took it and the result showed I was not a morning person (lark) or a night person (owl). I knew I was not a morning person. I can't function for at least an hour after I wake up.

Although I've always wanted to be a lark because they "have a mental edge, more quality white matter," I thought I may have been a combination of a lark and an owl, and a bit of a hummingbird, too. I researched and found that survey from 1973 and I still don't know what it means. But at the time it seemed important that I determine what kind of bird I was. Forty years later, when I looked back at that self-assessment, I think I have just adapted to life's demands. My world at times was a 24-hour operation. At the end of the day, or night, just as the self-assessment states, most owls, larks, and even hummingbirds, find a secure roost. Many of my colleagues have had to find a perch in each other. This is not just because we work at night, but because we are nurses.

I worried about driving and making sound decisions when I worked overnight. Most often, I had to return to work the next night, where I was required to be on high alert and make split-second, life-or-death decisions. I look back at pictures sometimes to find what looks like a propped-up mannequin, in a red outfit, eyes shut, snoring, right in the middle of the family celebration. I wondered why they always had to take the picture.

I was very nervous because I had learned in nursing school that staying awake all night changes your cortisol levels and causes "circadian misalignment." During my first five years, I worked the night shift occasionally, back when I did not have children. That was easy because I would come home and sleep twelve hours and go back to bed that same night, too. Later on, when I went back to nights after my last child was born, it was very difficult. My youngest went to kindergarten and told the teacher I did not work, I "just slept all the time."

Falling asleep mid-sentence is how I met a very good friend. While watching my son play baseball on a Saturday afternoon (after being awake 36 hours) I remember talking to another mother and then ending my thoughts. She woke me up so I would not fall of the bleachers. I apologized and told her I'd worked the night before. Her response was that she had worked last weekend. "Go sleep in the car, I'll watch your son," she told me. "I'll cheer him on," she promised, and I'm sure she did. This came with a deal: "Next weekend I'll sleep in the car and you watch my son."

Thirty years later, we are still good friends. She's still that kind of person, too. She has given me much more than a shoulder to sleep on during all these years. I'll be forever grateful that she's my friend and I'm hers. I know both of us have many, many stories about working nights as nurses.

Working nights is never healthy, especially as a nurse. One morning, my colleague almost made it home after a mandatory sixteen-hour night shift. She turned the corner to her street and does not remember anything after that. She woke up in her car, which had flipped upside down and ended up in her side yard. Stories like this that make you think that it does not matter when you sleep, day or night. Even for night owls, being a nurse on the night shift is hard. I do know one thing, though—I suspect she is a not a night owl, but more of a lark; she's loyal, and I guess you could say she can fly upside down.

The holidays can be difficult for those who work at night. If you are a nurse on the night shift, you are obligated to work either the night before the holiday or come into work at 11: 00 p.m. the night of the holiday. This includes the "eve" holidays. Some kids had to wait until Mom got home to see if Santa came. Others watched as Mom came home from work, got all dressed up, and fell asleep during the celebrations. Working against my natural sleep cycle caused fatigue, which at times worsened my mood. I know it diminished my cognitive abilities, and made me more vulnerable to sickness.

Operating room nurses don't necessarily work the night shift. In very large trauma centers, this may be the norm because all three shifts have a full complement of staff. Working in a small community hospital is quite different. Our shifts frequently consist of taking "call" at the conclusion of our day. Being on-call during the week consists of being readily available until the next morning. On weekends, the on-call requirements may extend to 48 hours of availability. Some days, we don't get to go home at all. The mandatory overtime statutes do not apply to operating room nurses. We would get in the habit of laying out our clothes before going to bed just in case we get called in during the middle of the night.

When that dreaded call comes, we rush into work, often with minimal rest periods, knowing that the slightest delay can have catastrophic outcomes for the patient; we know the patient with the ruptured aortic aneurysm doesn't have a second to spare. We are well aware of the obligations that come the next day, even after being on call through the night.

OR nurses know that a patient's surgery should not be cancelled because we happened to be on call all night. There are times when we miss family functions and school activities because of being on call. I am retired now, but after more than forty years of taking call, my heart still pounds when the phone rings in the middle of the night. But I wouldn't have changed careers for the world. I made a difference.

> *Extraordinary nurses enable patients to defy the odds every day. Nurses also marshal that same spirit to make it through fundraisers, blizzards, and all manner of natural and man-made crises. As with other personnel who work through difficult times, nurses know that there is perhaps no greater glue than spending a half-awake night on a row of cots with colleagues desperate for rest.*

I must admit I can be defiant when I am told something can't be done. My colleagues and I were aware that many of the children in the neighborhood surrounding our hospital were in need of coats and hats. Local agencies were desperately looking for donations. I suggested a cupcake war to raise money. I was told we would not raise money making cupcakes and that this would not really be a war. Bernard Shaw once said: "People who say it cannot be done, should not interrupt those who are doing it." I happen to think he was right.

Later that week, just about every employee brought in two dozen cupcakes. We raised $1,454.66 in four hours. We sold every cupcake. The social worker for the hospital told us that every child in the neighborhood would get a coat and a hat that year. Don't ever underestimate the commitment of a nurse investing in something much larger than herself. There is a certain pleasure in defying the odds, but beyond that, it was satisfying to support colleagues supporting their community.

It wouldn't have occurred to us not to go to work on January 9, 1978, or February 6, 1978, or during any other storm. It didn't matter that we saw a record ice storm or a record snowfall of more than forty inches of snow. In some areas it was more than four inches per hour. It didn't matter that some of my colleagues were even expecting children—we got there by snowmobile, state police, or police and fire escort. For these particular storms, we stayed at work more than five days, away from families, friends, and the rest of the world. It wasn't because we were martyrs, or because we failed to worry about our own personal safety. We worked out of a matter of duty, so to speak. For me, it was the feeling I got just being part of it all. During these blizzards and other emergencies, there was also a storm going on INSIDE the hospital. There were command centers and departments organizing to make sure there were adequate amounts of food, water, and other supplies for patients and staff. At first, the food seems great. After a few days the supply is usually sandwiches and bottled water. Both were appreciated nonetheless.

The most rewarding part was after the storm was over. Walking outside, you had to cover your eyes from the sun after five days inside the hospital. Waving goodbye and saying "great job" to one another, we would trudge to our cars only to see them already cleaned off. The four feet of snow would somehow be gone, the car unburied and shoveled out. Sometimes you could guess who had helped, but sometimes you did not know. There would be notes of thanks on your windshield and smiley faces on pieces of paper slipped into the door handle. As much as you want to be with your family during these times to make sure they are safe, there's something special about knowing how much you're needed and appreciated because you weren't.

To some, storm days will be remembered by the number of feet of snow on the ground, the speed of the wind, how many trees came down, or the days without electricity. But they are remembered differently by those of us who know what the storm is like on the inside. Now, when I'm not at work during a storm, my mind is always on those that are. I know how tired they are and that they are sleeping on cots and eating cold sandwiches. I know administration is counting the bottles of fresh water and constantly re-evaluating the disaster board. I appreciate every one of them.

You haven't really bonded with your colleagues until you have stayed at work for an extended length of time due to a blizzard, storm, or other emergency. For a few hours, you are assigned to steal some sleep on stretchers and cots lined up in the auditorium before returning to work. There is a fear of falling asleep and snoring or doing something even worse next to the nurse you have to work with tomorrow. But at least you're all in it together. Each one of you prays that the next shift is able to "make it in" so you may "make it out." If it lasts longer than most of you can tolerate, even the free food that the administration brings up from the kitchen doesn't cut it.

I played a minute role in the attempt to decrease the incidence of Ebola in the United States. There were many others surrounding me who contributed much more. But that time in my career (and even my small contribution) are so memorable to me. During the Ebola outbreak, I was with a fellow graduate student who was originally from Liberia. She was working closely with friends and relatives, giving countless informational sessions to them, and encouraging them to report symptoms and recent travel even when they were completely afraid of doing so.

The hospital I was working at was chosen as the spot where potential patients would be transported. We were collaborating with the most educated epidemiologists in the world from the Centers for Disease Control and Prevention (CDC). I remember being totally impressed with the knowledge of the epidemiologists I worked with. Of course, none of them had ever seen Ebola. Still, their contributions to the development of screenings and processes were incredible to witness. Overall, this was an honor but it was also devastating. I worked with the most dedicated nurses at the time. Still, being asked to develop the plans for this was overwhelming.

This was an experience I will never forget. Advances in technology, education, and science have made our profession a global one. When diseases and human beings collide, sometimes resulting in an epidemic, nurses always step forward. This time, I learned that when we take that step, we're never walking alone.

The work of nursing has changed with the times in response to internal and external forces. Yet nursing is (and has always been) about teamwork. In some instances, that team is changed by something global like a shortage; at other times, a nurse responds to the changing idea of a family.

In the twenty years I have been a bedside nurse, I am grateful to see how the definition of family has changed and the impact this has had on our practice. The term "family" now reflects diversity. I have seen how our professional understanding of this determines how effective we will be overall. Family structures not only impact the family as a whole, but the health of the individuals in it. To be effective in teaching health and wellness, we must understand the influence family members have on the patterns of health. There is no doubt that the family is also the patient, and this must influence our practice.

In the spring of 2008, I was called to the Human Resources department at my hospital. This could have been devastating, but I was nearly confident it was not. I would later learn that I wasn't the first one to be approached, but I was the last. The director of Human Resources asked me if I had a U.S. Passport. I did not. They needed someone to travel to the Middle East and recruit nurses. They asked if I knew where I would be going. I did not. I soon got ahold of a passport, but also a map.

Two weeks later, I was on my way to the Middle East. After more than twenty hours in an airplane, I met some of the most passionate nurses I will ever know. I had been given instructions from Human Resources, including what questions to ask and how to determine competence. If you knew me at all, you would know I was not going to comply with the questions they had picked. While I considered these questions important, the answers would not reflect what we needed. I am being asked to decide on "the best fit" for our organization. I didn't believe that I alone could determine this with the questions I was given to ask. Besides, I was changing these interviewees' lives dramatically. How do I choose the "best fit" for someone who is willing to travel more than 6,500 miles for a job? How do I choose the "best fit" from among a group of people willing to move from a place where it is 100 degrees at midnight to a place that has three feet of snow on the ground?

It turns out I could only select twenty-five out of the more than one hundred people I interviewed. This made the original interview questions even more obsolete. The process of choosing was overwhelming. But by this time, I had decided to approach the interviewing in a different way, with my questions. I asked each candidate to tell me about a time when they felt they made a difference in someone's life. I asked about experiences, not skills. I knew that with the right training, anyone can calculate a mean arterial blood pressure. Talking to these women, I was looking for something different.

One nurse told me how she cared for a young woman with Guillain-Barre syndrome. She apologized upfront for her command of English, but I didn't really have any trouble. I understood her perfectly when she explained that her patient had given birth while paralyzed. This patient began walking again just as her own daughter did, one year later. She told me "this was more than five years ago," but I could tell it was as if it had happened yesterday. For a brief moment, she stared into space. I knew what she was doing in that moment because I've had them, too. She was remembering the patient's face at the exact moment that she realized she just might get well. Her command of English didn't matter at all. Her stories were my stories. Institutions responded to the nursing shortage in the United States in different ways. At the time I was sent to Dubai, the nursing shortage was significantly affecting every acute and chronic care facility. Many administrators and human resource departments were forced to do something unconventional. In a way, I was, too. This was an experience I'll never forget.

A lot of my colleagues will claim they work within an interdisciplinary team. This method of care has been shown through research to be the most beneficial for optimal patient outcomes. No one in healthcare would disagree. Working in silos has never been shown to decrease infections, fall rates, or any other hospital acquired condition. There is often a lot of talk, and a lot of research, but I will just say I was part of a team that proved it.

How do you get fifty healthcare workers, including pharmacists, intensivists, registered nurses, social workers, and respiratory therapists to meet and academically discuss clostridium difficile (ahem, C Diff) therapies on a Saturday morning? It's not as difficult as you might imagine when people understand the stakes. The staff believed that if they were more informed about a condition that threatened their patients in their unit, the incidence could be decreased. It was the same for other topics, including carbon monoxide poisoning. That meeting came after a family in our community suffered from it. Working alongside professionals that show how much they care about patient outcomes is one part of the puzzle.

Another element is the power of lateral support, which has a tremendous impact. I think being a member of a healthcare team is just that. Nursing colleagues do not always wear the "RN" in big red font on their badge. They wear PT, OT, PharmD, MD, PA, SW and many more. Alone, you're only a small piece of the puzzle, just one person assessing, diagnosing, and intervening, all in an effort to give the best care to the patient. But together, with the right people, you're the whole box of the pieces and the glue.

Not all relationships between nurses are positive. In some instances, lateral violence significantly impacts how nurses function in their roles. Any examination of collegiality would be incomplete without a look at this issue, which by definition is the absence of collegial behavior. Similarly, those in nursing "are not immune to disease, including addiction," as one contributor writes, and this too deserves inspection.

There is research identifying lateral violence in nursing as far back as forty years ago. Along with this research are strategies to avoid, identify, and eliminate it. Researchers speculate as to why it exists, and a lot of research states that it simply should not exist among professionals. Others have developed theories to explain and predict it. Still, lateral violence has been documented as a prevalent problem in nursing.

Although I have studied the theories about lateral violence and some of the best solutions to predict and avoid it, when it came to being a victim, it didn't matter that I understood the theories. It made me physically sick. It also made me leave a role I loved. I had a colleague explain it to me this way: "You're feeling the effects of the Kryptonite." She went on, "I have felt it, too." I thought a lot about this analogy. While I was feeling so guilty about being affected by the bullying, I forgot to use my superpowers to face it. "That's the Kryptonite," she said. This seemed so simple. I asked if that was how she faced it. She told me instead of thinking about the fact that it should not happen, think about it always being a possibility, at least from some people. "Then you'll be ready...ready for the Kryptonite." I was able to recover somewhat from being treated unfairly.

I'm not sure about "always being ready" for it, though. I still believe it's not professional and shouldn't be tolerated. But in order to be able to care for others, I think we do need that superpower at times, in part to defend against the Kryptonite. It can be so fast moving and unexpected. This philosophy worked for me. She then suggested that being self-deprecating helps. I'll have to look that up after our shift, I thought, I know it sounds like something else entirely but I'm sure she's not talking about defecation here. Our worlds are sometimes filled with "look-alike, sound-alikes," I thought. What I do remember is this, her laughter and her line: "Just call me Lois Lane," when I thanked her.

We know that we, as nurses, are not immune to disease, including addiction. It is difficult to discuss; it is more difficult to report, but we must. Our obligation is to the patient. The opioid epidemic knows no boundaries and makes hostages of many who innocently become victims after being prescribed an opioid for pain management. Some people (some of whom others are unaware of) have successfully completed diversion programs and continue to have exceptional nursing careers, just as many of our patients have experienced that success. What is important is to re-establish trust. The patient must have trust in the nurse; the nurse must trust the colleague; the victims need a system they can trust to help them.

> *Much of a nurse's on-the-job training comes from colleagues and mentors. A few people in particular have stood out for these nurses who have been inspired to write about the leaders who enabled them to thrive.*

I have had the privilege of working with the best and for the best. In the 1970s, my first nurse leader (we called her the head nurse, a term that has been eliminated) was the epitome of the nursing school graduate. At just five feet, she stood tall in the starched uniform, perfectly polished shoes, pins, and cap. She had it all on every day. She would not stand for anything but the best for her patients; that ward was her life, her pride.

I was caught one day not warming up the lotion in my hand before a backrub. She quietly called me over and squirted it down my back, ice cold. I never did that again. She demanded the best on her ward and everyone delivered. The physicians all wanted their patients on "her" ward. It was hers, but not one of us minded, we were proud to work there. I don't know why it never occurred to us at the time to think of it as our ward.

It was about four years later when everyone noticed her obvious abdomen. She was still fairly young, so was it possible? It couldn't be. She was a tiny lady, by all descriptions. But her abdomen grew by the week. It was lymphoma. Her colleagues swarmed like bees. The care she was given was quiet, efficient, and impeccable. Her privacy was never compromised. We protected her. She was cared for by the best, the same nurses she had demanded the best from. I don't think she ever suffered. In the end, the nurses that she demanded so much from gave so much back to her.

I spent about thirty years working for a nurse who knew the definition of leadership. She had a grasp of critical care beyond all others and most importantly, she understood family. She was the member of management I would admire for being so real. She treated everyone that worked for her the exact same way, which was respectfully. I never knew a day I regretted working for her; she referred to the Intensive Care as "our unit." She involved you in making decisions about the unit and the patients, and it made you accountable for the mistakes. She holds herself up for the same accountability that we have. She is supportive.

This woman is the nurse in the hospital that all of the other leaders look to. I consider her the best nursing leader I have ever known, not because she always agreed with me, but because she knew I really cared, and recognized my faults. She never failed to congratulate me or thank me if I helped a colleague. Thank you, Ginny, for being such a successful woman. Thank you for being in my life.

Although nursing was my dream, there were many obstacles that forced me to take the scenic route toward my quest. My parents both worked hard but couldn't afford to pay for college. During my senior year of high school, I attempted to join the Air Force as a means to reach my goal. Because I was only seventeen, my parents refused to give consent. "The military is no place for a young girl," they protested. Still determined, I heard about a program at a local hospital that offered training in addition to a stipend for those interested in becoming a surgical technician. I quickly applied and was ecstatic to be accepted. I successfully completed the nine-month program and became a surgical technician, a title I held for twenty-two years.

I loved my job, but still held on to my dream of becoming a registered nurse. Many of my colleagues encouraged me to further my education. One nurse in particular was relentless. She convinced me that I had so much more to offer. She even took me to the community college to register for my first class, the first step in pursuing my dream. She then guided me throughout the transition of realizing my dream.

The hospital that I worked at offered tuition reimbursement, which made acquiring my associate's degree in nursing financially manageable. While working full-time and attending classes two nights per week and on Saturdays, I completed my prerequisites and applied to the evening nursing program. Once enrolled in the nursing program, I was working full-time and doing my clinicals every other four-day weekend. This made finding time to study challenging but not impossible. The doctors grilled me on anatomy during surgical cases. Nurses reinforced what I read in books.

I completed the curriculum and clinical requirements, graduating in 1993. My colleague was once again by my side, this time attending my pinning ceremony. As a graduation gift she gave me a membership to the Association of Operating Room Nurses (AORN). She then insisted that I become certified as quickly as time allowed (CNOR). I still continue both the membership and my certification into my retirement.

Even with all of this, my colleague still wasn't satisfied. "You need to get your BSN," she insisted." I loved being in school and excelled, graduating Magna Cum Laude. We have been friends for many years and I have always looked to her for guidance. She has never disappointed me and I am forever grateful that she came into my life. Nursing wasn't my job, it was my passion. The path was difficult. I would have never succeeded without Joanne.

For those of us who are older, the image of a nurse is different. We think of the Barbie doll nurse—the figure with the cap, starched white uniform, clinic shoes, and a chart in hand. We probably never think of the nurses who spend their time behind the doors that read "Restricted Area-Operating Room Personnel Only."

This territory, which is foreign to most, is a critical area of nursing practice that is often forgotten. How unfortunate that the only exposure to the surgical arena is most likely a day of observation during clinicals. Long gone are the days when an operating room rotation was part of the curriculum. Perhaps this can explain why there is such a shortage of operating room nurses. Though many years have passed since I began my nursing career, I will always remember one of my instructors telling me, "I hope you don't plan on working in the OR. That's not nursing!" As a student, although I was highly insulted, I didn't dare confront her ignorance about the role of an operating room nurse.

As a surgical technician who had worked in the field for many years before becoming a nurse, I had deep admiration for the OR nurses I worked with and was eager to become one of them. It takes many months of additional education and training after completing nursing school to be able to function as a novice nurse in this specialty. Because there are so many different specialties to master, it also takes years to become proficient.

My instructor, like many others, assumed that the role of the OR nurse is charting and mostly technical. I am sure that she never saw the OR nurse in action. During an emergency, we can do a head-to-toe assessment in minutes. We address psychological needs, provide education, and hold the hands of patients during the scariest moments of their lives. Even though we are behind a mask, our eyes speak volumes. When patients ask what my role is as an OR nurse, I tell them the RN has many duties. The most important one for me, however, is being your voice when you don't have one. It is my responsibility to assure that all the necessary protocols and procedures that keep you safe are followed. I am your advocate when you're asleep.

One of my nursing school professors stands out. She taught the maternity, public health, and community health courses. She went above and beyond the classroom setting. She seemed to be the only professor we had that truly cared about what students had to say. If there was a problem, she wanted to hear our concerns and advocated for us. She also encouraged us to stand up for ourselves. The advice she gave us was wise and comforting. She had such a kind personality that it was easy to go to her for anything. Her door was always open and her ears were ready to listen. To have a professor like that definitely helped throughout all of the stress and anxiety of nursing school.

Nurses take care of each other; they share their stories. As I sit having lunch with my dear friend of more than thirty years, I have never been more aware that this is true. I only see my friend in the summer now, because she spends her winters in warmer weather. I tell her that I'm writing a story about when I was in nursing school. It hurts to think about that time in my life, but it's so important to acknowledge how my friend supported me.

This friend tells me she didn't plan on being a nurse, but when her job was eliminated in the rubber factory, she needed to find another way to support her children. It was the biggest factory of its kind in the world at the time. It wasn't needed anymore after WWII. When she found out it was closing, she was given a choice: hairdressing school or nursing school. Two of the women chose nursing and she was among them.

Without even having a high school diploma, she was determined. Donned in a navy-blue sweater, white shoes, and white stockings, she studied endlessly. Within one year she proudly wore the LPN cap and the initials. She reminisced, "I was respected when I got the job as an LPN ... I remember learning about the Stryker beds, and eventually being the one everyone relied on to use it." She admits to taking so much pride in the care she gave.

I look at her with admiration. I agree with her, without saying it, because it still hurts. She did take pride in her care. I know this personally. I was months from finishing nursing school myself when she proved she took pride in the care she gave. I was losing my mother and I wanted to quit nursing school. She gave me the strength to stay and helped me to care for my mother when I was losing her, despite having her own burdens from the war. Some would say that a good friend would help you and support you even if they were not a nurse. I suppose that's true. But I believe it's because we are both nurses that we can just look at each other and know exactly what to say and do at the right time.

It has been many years since she talked me into staying in nursing school, back when my world was falling apart. Yet I'll never forget how she supported me. She was right when she said, "I take pride in the care I give." We are both retired now. We talk often but see each other much less. We talk about being operating room nurses, our families, and the usual. I don't believe it's a cliché that some people come into your life for a reason. I know for a fact it's because we are nurses that we know how to care for each other. Thank you, Maggie.

Mentorship has long been described and studied in nursing practice, mostly as a framework. The attributes of the mentor have also been studied. The concept has been used concurrently with "preceptorship," "orienteer," and "supervisor." This story is not about an attempt to describe or explain a mentor relationship; it's simply a reflection on how it felt to hear that I have been a mentor. There have been many times in my career that I don't think I realized I was being a mentor; I just thought that what I was doing was an opportunity to enhance someone else's career. But the recipients have used the words "great mentor." That correlation has never been described in studies about mentorship.

As someone who believes in lifelong learning, but also someone who realizes that life gets in the way, I have encouraged so many to pursue education. I also stressed that the timing must be perfect. It's not always a great time to try and achieve a master's degree with certain other responsibilities. More than several times I have felt successful, however. One time I was asked to pin a colleague as she was handed her BSN. I cried during the pinning, partially because I know the obstacles she had to endure and partially due to the simple fact she had asked me to pin her.

Another time I heard that I had done something that changed a career path. Initially, I had just thought it would be enriching to have one of my colleagues witness me reading, discussing, and signing a master's degree thesis. Later, he said it was a highlight of his career. Mentoring, encouraging, and supportive behavior should be the basis for nursing practice itself. Mentoring means being an advocate—not just for our patients—but each other.

The dining room was whirring with the sounds of sewing machines working at full capacity. The kitchen was full of ironing boards and attendants ready for the next swatch of fabric. I will admit that I avoided those two stations, but for good reason. First, I loved to cook, and second, I knew the self-proclaimed "project manager" was over there and I knew nothing about sewing. So instead I called out "first supper," mimicking our life at the hospital. We weren't there for the meal, however.

We had gathered to assemble a homemade quilt for someone very special to us. Earlier this year, like all of the other years, we had talked about what to give our manager for Christmas. We discussed the usual suspects : a restaurant gift card, briefcase, special pen, or sweater for the dogs she loved so much. Someone suggested a homemade quilt, and even though it was met with skepticism and many remarks of "I don't sew," we all thought it was a great idea to give her something personal.

We each designed a fabric square that reflected our bond with our manager. Because she and I shared the bond of graduating from the same nursing school, and both loved golf, my square to her was just that. Of course, we all felt our own squares were the best. We disagreed on that point, but never on the discussion of Ginny being the best for each one of us. This was so typical of critical care nurses. The "project manager" watched with an eagle eye to make sure the squares were all aligned. As critical care nurses, we would not have wanted it any other way. Just like all of our IV tubing, they had to be lined up and labeled perfectly; "not like some of the other units," someone commented.

We felt such pride when our manager opened that quilt at the Christmas party. We were proud of the sewing, the ironing, and the great meal that helped us make it. Just like any day in the Intensive Care Unit, we knew we could not have done it all alone. We appreciated not only the camaraderie that day, but more importantly, the honor of working with such a great role model. We knew the bond between us was as interwoven as the stiches on the quilt.

I am honored to have known, worked for, and been a friend of Rosemary. The first time I met her in August 2002, I knew I had met an extraordinary person. She was brilliant and I always felt I learned something after speaking with her. Rosemary was an advocate for the patient and felt nurses and physicians needed to work collaboratively for patients to have the best outcomes. Her passion was contagious and we always gave our all for her. When she was diagnosed with cancer, I was devastated. Even though she is no longer with us, she is always with me.

In their communities, many nurses might be known as caregivers or role models. Some take their care for others to the next level by becoming involved in advocacy.

Nurses fulfill many different roles. I have always felt that the most important role of the nurse is to be the patient advocate. My written job evaluations have always reflected that belief. Another, less contemplated role is that of political activist. During my long career, I have testified before the House of Representatives and Senate in our state many times. These representatives rely on testimony from the experts in the field of nursing to guide their legislative decisions. My testimony was educational, providing insights into the nursing profession that were foreign to those who create our laws. During this testimony, law makers were allowed to ask questions about how the public will be impacted by their decision.

It gives me such a sense of accomplishment to follow the progress of a bill presented by a legislature. That bill will go through multiple hearings and votes to eventually become law. Sometimes it can take years to accomplish. In the end, I know that my voice has made a difference. I have written to congressmen and the President of the United States about issues that impact healthcare or the nursing profession. Some of those letters have received a written response. On two occasions, I have also been granted a personal meeting to discuss an agenda. If we, the experts, don't tell of our concerns, how will they know?

So much of being a nurse revolves around the shift—the time spent at work. But the spirit of nursing is something that stays with you long after you clock out. It is something you can only feel after being in the practice of the profession and as one writer suggests, it is something that cannot leave you.

We are taught the basics of nursing practice in the very first lectures in nursing. We learn the scope, the standards, and even the definition of practice. Roles in nursing are also clearly defined by the professors. I felt I was well prepared to promote, optimize, and prevent illness and injury. I understood the concept of nursing as an art and a science and what makes me a professional—that specific body of knowledge.

What I was not prepared for was this: the collegiality I would feel. My colleagues came from every nursing program in the state. They graduated with varying grades, degrees, and scores on their NCLEX. No matter which shift I rotate to or what unit I float to, I have found a colleague I can rely on. I know my colleagues are there for me and for their patients, the primary concern we all share. I have been an RN for less than one year. I am a novice, as Patricia Benner would say. I was taught that realizing I'm a novice is important in understanding critical thinking and reflection in practice. Those were just words a year ago, back when I had to memorize Benner's Novice to Expert. But they are not just words anymore now that I have applied them. I can't wait for the day I am experienced enough to be the role model my colleagues have been to me. I am so proud to be called a nurse.

Your colleagues are in a role with you. They don't go to work, they function in a role. It is one of the most profound. The role of a nurse is life affecting, it's always there, in you, even when you are not functioning in it. With that in mind, when I decided to leave bedside nursing and go into teaching, I found myself wondering if I was still a nurse. I wanted to believe that I was, more than anything, but there were doubts circling around my head. Then this happened.

A small group of students stayed after class to discuss a case study. Their questions were typical of nursing students in their first semester: are vital signs subjective? When do you re-evaluate? After answering their questions, it was my turn to ask a few of them. I inquired as to how their first two classes in nursing were going so far. Answering quickly, it was apparent they had already discussed this. They all turned around to make sure that their classmates had left the classroom. Then, one of the students said, "I hope you understand this when I tell you how I feel." "Of course," I replied, encouraging her to continue. She went on to say, "when you explained the nursing process last week, and we actually got to do a care plan, I felt happy." She had always wanted to be a nurse, but didn't know what the role was truly about, just that "I knew it would make me happy." Her classmates nodded. "I feel the same way," they said. I acknowledged their feelings, adding that I, too, felt the same. On the way out, I overheard one of them say to the other, "I knew she would understand what I meant." I am still a nurse.

Chapter Five

As We Know It

*Kristine Batty, Kelly Baxter, Denise Bezila,
Patricia Bonzagni, Jeannine Borozny, Rebecca Carley,
Linda Del Vecchio-Gilbert, Robert Desrosiers,
Pam DiMascio, Donna Dupuis, Lucille Ferrer,
Leiah Gallagher, Marla Goulart,
Donna Horrocks, Lisa Johnson,
Rebecca L. Jones, Rachel Jones,
Elaine Joyal, Linda Lambert,
Kristina Lambert, Mary Lavin,
Shelley MacDonald, Alisha Mal,
Michelle Mallon, Colleen Moynihan,
Deborah Myers, Stacie Nunziato,
Ellen O'Rourke, Anabela O'Shea,
Darlene Noret, Kathleen O'Connell, Angela
Quarters, Deborah Quirk, Elizabeth Raposa,
Barbara Saleeba, Cathy Schwartz, Linda Tierney,
Karen Treloar, Cynthia Votto,
Rosemary Walker, Virginia Wilcox,
Dianna Wantoch, Karen Zarlenga*

This final chapter includes meditations on what nursing has meant to each individual who contributed to the book. These short and elegant reflections speak for themselves.

For nurses of a certain age, there was the Barbie nurse, Cherry Ames, and Marcus Welby. I often wonder what the next generation's influence will be.

Although my career evolved from bedside nursing to advanced practice, I continued to see the fundamentals of the professional role. Over 20 years, I see the influence of social, historical, political, and economic changes on nursing practices. Included in these changes are evolving roles of nursing and more opportunities to influence health behaviors. But fundamentally, we are all providers of care, in direct care, acute care, community, respite care and much more.

To me, nursing means learning, research, teamwork and the sacred opportunity to connect with the patients and their families when they are most vulnerable.

My career has been wonderful. I liken my career to this: it has been a great marriage, nursing and I. When I've been down, it's always been there. It has nurtured and supported me and my family. I have given much to it- but it has given me so much more. Thank you, nursing, I love you.

We practice in roles—as educators, administrators, researchers. Because of this, there is always the importance of understanding demographic changes, such as the rural to urban shifts, in both chronic and acute care, for any of these roles. There is even more importance in knowing the influence we have on quality for vulnerable populations, the medically underserved.

My nursing career has meant more to me than only caring for patients. It has meant learning about more global and universal concepts, some which have come to impact me as a person. I learned about "the graying of America" and although I conceptually understand the unique needs of the older adult, I am like most people and felt like that would not be me, not ever. But I have felt the impact of ageism and it is not pleasant. The positive result of this is that I am fortunate to be in a position to influence other nurses that ageism is not acceptable. Perhaps when this plea comes from a colleague who they have seen grow with them, it is considered sound. I truly appreciate my colleagues for not ever thinking I may be too old to understand nursing.

In giving, we are given.

We earn our own reputations. We are all in our own generations of the profession. We should never be afraid to welcome new ideas, growth. It doesn't matter who generates the new knowledge as long as we share.

Although personal situations often impact many of my decisions as a person, personal influences only impact my profession in one situation: respect for personal dignity.

I believe that trust has to be important. It's the nurse-patient relationship. I believe because of their extreme vulnerability, patients and their families need this mechanism, allowing them the ability to trust another human being to communicate the truth, allowing them to be vulnerable, and to understand, is the most important aspect of regaining autonomy in the setting of critical illness.

The experience of vulnerability can be felt in our personal lives without any warning. We, as human beings, can be affected by vulnerability at any given time. In the intensive care unit population, both patients and families can be affected by vulnerability, and their autonomy can be compromised. I think vulnerability is one of the most important concepts for nurses to understand, especially in the ICU.

As a nurse, even though you understand the physiological reasons that disease impacts humans, it is so stressful to witness your loved one become debilitated by disease; unable to communicate, physically move, eat.

I will never forget the day I had to leave my critically ill mother in the ICU. I was so happy to know she was in very capable hands, my colleagues' hands. As a nurse, I know how important empathy is. As a daughter, I know I felt it that day.

My patients: I looked to them as individuals who were courageous and inspiring.

With endless appreciation, I thank every patient who has touched my life, providing me with strength, wisdom and guidance. Their lives have touched mine in ways unimaginable.

How do you find peace with some of the deaths you see? Even with debriefing it is so difficult.

End of life care is one of the most important times you can display advocacy for a patient. You should always feel emotion at the end of someone's life—always. It is time to not be a nurse when you don't feel a loss.

I will never forget the heartache and anguish of a family who has lost a child. I felt it myself and I don't even love that child.

There are the patients who are so critically ill that almost no one expects them to survive. But with the team of disciplines who are diligent and relentless in their efforts to save this patient, the patient survives and comes back to visit when they are well. That is the ultimate in happiness. The list could go on and on.

There was the family of a young mother who sustained a sudden cardiac arrest. Their desire to donate her organs so others may have the chance to live took the highest level of support, compassion and caring.

I love every aspect of the nurse practitioner role and continue in my role as "neighborhood nurse" …there are so many pictures of body parts, rashes, and questions on my cell phone. Was this the first tele-health?

I feel like my children were more educated and aware of safety because I worked in emergency nursing. They never rode their bicycles without sneakers on and never rode their scooters without a helmet. I took it to the extreme. You WILL lose all of your toenails and will NEVER walk again. I don't regret it.

I think being a nurse definitely impacted the way I raised my children. They learned quickly what was an emergency was and what was not. They learned respect for my role in the hospital. That meant I could not be disturbed unless it was absolutely necessary. I once overheard one of them telling their friends that "the house had to be on fire to call my Mom at work."

I have been fortunate enough to advance my education in nursing. Taking leadership classes and studying the characteristics of leaders was so relevant to what I had lived for years. It's true that leaders are found at the bedside, in administration, and beyond. It's not the title, it's the attributes. Staff members identify with leaders even without the title or their access to the nursing leadership meetings. They are approachable, acting as mentors and role models. What I learned was that the best leaders are visible, have integrity, and at least some clinical competence.

As an RN, your knowledge of the political system can contribute to the quality of health practices in nursing. I have had the opportunity to testify several times on health-related issues, such as mandatory overtime, safe staffing, and years ago, the use of latex. I have also testified as a consumer of healthcare. It is important for all nurses to have a voice in healthcare. So often decision making does not involve us, and we are at the forefront of the patient arena. We are not just constituents, we are advocates and caregivers and we are often in the best possession of knowledge that can protect the most vulnerable. I am proud of the influences I have had legislatively.

The profession of nursing has been one my life's greatest gifts. It has been an honor to be someone's nurse. My life is different, changed, and honored by all those who my eyes have met, whose hands I have touched, and whose hearts invited to me to be present.

Upon completing my 40th year in the profession of nursing, I have come to realize that this profession is enriched by those who require care, those that are learning, and those who face adversity. I learned that patients are the ultimate teachers. They are the very teachers that shaped my life as a young nurse, mother, nurse educator and fellow colleague.

To me, nursing is totally about making the connection with your patient. The patient must feel confident in you, know you care about them, and trust you. Without that connection there can be a tendency to drift away from what is most important, the patient. As I reflect upon my nursing career, I remember many special patients.

The support and camaraderie I have found in nursing is invaluable to me and I am fortunate to have a career that I love.

Today, I have been a nurse for more than 47 years. I still work full-time in critical care. I look forward to semi-retirement in a few years. But I am happy to realize so many things about nursing. The compassion, respect, and devotion I feel for my patients is what nurses them back to better health. I make a difference in their recovery. As long as I can speak and think, I will have shoulders for my patients to lean on. It's this that makes me respect myself, feel proud of what I do, and who I have become. This is not just a job.

I was afraid that I wouldn't feel like a nurse if I were to leave the patient's bedside and go into teaching. My very first week, I realized how wrong I was. I'm able to mentor and set expectations for these students about their career. I find it sometimes even more rewarding to emulate what success looks like in nursing. I don't feel as though this is boastful, it's really a chance to role model. Teaching has allowed me to discuss some of the more difficult aspects of nursing and give guidance to groups of young men and women who are just as passionate as I am. Teaching allows me to reflect on my experiences as a nurse. Some of the scenarios I'm able to use are recent, some in the distant past. I realize that what I have to offer is invaluable. Without these experiences students in nursing are only learning tasks. Although these tasks are important, to me, it's really the art of nursing that makes us unique as professionals.

I'm not sure if my nursing career follows me, or is within me. I know it's central to how I think. My family knows I'm what they call "global" about it. If I am on vacation, I have to interrogate the locals about their healthcare system. It's not to validate what I think is wrong with ours, it's to gain perspective, I tell them. I have to plan precisely—if it's an island adventure, an isolated area, I need to know about their prevention practices, immunizations, and Zika rates, for example. At times, I need more intense questioning about nursing care practices and protocols. If we're international, my family understands it could be the perfect time to discuss socialized medicine vs. private. It's truly just scientific information I'm after, I assure them. I'm not sure they are convinced it's always necessary, or truly just information that I need. I think it can make them a little uneasy. Nurses are needed all over the world, and often I'm offered a job immediately; this also makes some travel companions nervous.

Looking back at my life, I feel so lucky to have chosen nursing as my profession! Growing up, there were not as many career choices for women as there are today. Many of my friends wanted to be teachers or secretaries. Only a handful expressed an interest in nursing. As for me, I really did not know how I could make a difference. In fact, when I really began to lean toward a nursing career, my guidance counselor discouraged me because I was not very strong in the sciences. But I had gotten a taste of the hospital setting by working as a volunteer (candy striper). As I sat with patients and helped to comfort them, I knew what I wanted. I applied to nursing school despite the objection of my guidance counselor, was accepted, and have never regretted that decision.

To me, nursing means learning and research and teamwork and the sacred opportunity to connect with the patients and their families when they are most vulnerable. There are also endless opportunities available to nurses. There are nursing specialties such as emergency nursing, critical care nursing, surgical nursing, pediatric nursing, and obstetrical nursing. There are roles for staff nurses, managers, directors, chief nursing officers and nurse practitioners. There are certainly challenges along the way, but I can tell you that I would choose the same career today as I chose many years ago.

When I look back over my 50 years in nursing, I am amazed by all the advances that I've had the pleasure of being part of. I can only imagine what the future of nursing will bring!

Humility.

Chapter Six

As We Remember It

Many of us have experienced tremendous changes in nursing practice over the past half century. Our stories have shown us that despite all that shifts around us, we are never alone in this spirit of nursing. No matter where they practice, our colleagues have similar practices, challenges, and triumphs.

Looking back on our shared history has also reminded us of the global events where a professional nurse's presence was felt. This, too, is included in our shared spirit of nursing.

Nursing must be a dynamic field, always searching. We must focus on providing safe care for our patients. But in addition, we must provide safe environments for ourselves. Often, nurses have to focus on the day-to-day. But looking back and learning from our shared history, our legacies, is also important.

The nursing environment has changed since its early years as a profession. Yet we are still connected to our early leaders in our shared focus on the patient. Some suggest we should always reflect back on the Nightingales Pledge as core to our profession. Graduates of nursing programs continue to recite Florence Nightingale's words at the pinning ceremony.

Thus, in spite of all that has changed since Nightingale's day, across the world, new nurses can be found declaring that they will: "Practice the profession faithfully and with purity; do no harm; elevate the standard of the profession and be loyal to their work and devoted towards the welfare of their clients." The methods to accomplish the pledge have changed but the words are as relevant as ever.

What follows are a stream of thoughts on concrete changes in practice. Practitioners who have been at work for many years share their ideas on how nursing has evolved for the past half century or so. They also connect their local experiences to major world events and catastrophes. In all, these are final reflections on how the spirit of nursing has moved through generations of nurses throughout time.

In my years of nursing, I have seen many changes in the health care field. In other times, intravenous bottles were glass; there were no IV pumps. We "time taped" all our infusions and monitored the drip every hour. Johnnies had no snaps on the sleeve and all IV bottles had to be threaded through the sleeves. Creativity and new forms of technology have led to a much easier way of delivering IV medications and dispensing medications.

In the past, nurses always wore white uniforms; they had white dresses, white shoes, and stockings. We'd hope we wouldn't get stains on our uniforms or a run in our stockings. The distinction of the white uniform has faded. Nurses now wear many different colors and styles of uniforms. We wonder if clients are not always recognizing who is the nurse and who is the housekeeper. Nursing used to be considered a profession of females; the clear majority of nurses were women. Males were orderlies but not nurses. We are grateful more and more males are joining the nursing profession.

1970s

We thought about our nursing colleagues in 1974 during the "super outbreak" of hundreds of tornadoes in more than 15 states, and of course during the great blizzard that hit New England in the winter of 1978.

We remember...

In the 1970s, being diagnosed with a peptic ulcer meant bedrest for several weeks, sedatives, tranquilizers, calcium carbonate or aluminum hydroxide throughout the day and night. We would use anticholinergics to control gastric secretions. Belladonna was popular; I also remember Pro-Banthine. I remember the side effects these patients had, too. They were so thirsty. We used skim milk, alternating with cream, given po or through the nasogastric tube every hour. I'm not sure they healed well, but were discharged in a few weeks, at least without pain.

Although crash carts were starting to be introduced in the late 1960s, I never saw one as a student in 1971, or perhaps I was only focused on the Kardex and the Care Plan. There were no Code Blues, no ACLS, no post cardiac arrest care. As both myself and the science of resuscitation grew, I became so much more aware of our responsibility in not only knowing these new advancements, but looking forward to research that would enhance survival to an even greater degree.

Retrospectively, I think about all of the patients who were not fortunate enough to be alive during a time when patients receive multidisciplinary, evidenced based care.

I think back to a time when families were not included in the care plan. I think back to when the patient often did not have their loved one with them at one of the most difficult times of their life. But with that being said, I'm grateful this reflection makes me advocate for these situations to be different now.

In this time, rotating tourniquets were the therapeutic measure for heart failure. Three sphygmomanometer cuffs, applied to three out of four extremities, rotated every few minutes. It was a rigid schedule. It was often your sole responsibility and took the full attention of one nurse. Clysis was used as a therapy for patients in LTC. Hypodermoclysis needles were inserted subcutaneously to provide isotonic fluid replacement to older adults.

Back then, we smoked at the nurses' station. We smoked in the cafeteria, we smoked in the lounge, and during report. The monitors at the desk needed to be cleaned often due to the smoke film. We often had to empty ashtrays in the doctors' charting area.

We dispensed medications out of a system that resembled a cigarette machine. You selected the drug by the picture, pulled the knob and it fell below into a well. If you were the "medication nurse" you may have more than 40 little white cups with medications in them, placed in holes on a tray. The yellow "med card" had the patient's name and room number. What a contrast to presently having medication reconciliation and BCMA to prevent errors in the distribution of medications.

Everything seemed to be metal. There were metal bedpans, metal tracheostomy tubes, metal Kardexes, metal intravenous catheters.

So many patients had Latex urinary catheters in for weeks and nasogastric tubes in their noses, bigger than a garden hose.

During this time, we used heat lamps, Betadine and sometimes antacids and sugar to treat decubitus ulcers.

I remember using a hydrometer to measure urine specific gravity in the dirty utility room. It was made of glass; it was a cylindrical stem and a bulb weighted with mercury to make it float. I remember we shattered them a lot. We didn't think about reimbursement for the test or even quality control.

During client care we would not wear gloves to wash clients, empty urinary catheters, handle blood tubes.

1980s

> *We thought about our nursing colleagues caring for Barney Clark, the first person to have a permanent artificial heart implanted, and our colleagues doing the caring and being cared for during the deadliest nuclear power plant accident to date.*

We remember...

Gallbladder surgery would require a minimal 3-day hospital stay. The innovation of laparoscopic surgery dramatically reduced this expectation to that of an outpatient procedure. In conjunction with laparoscopic cameras, which can better visualize important structures through magnification, surgeons now use robotics to facilitate positive outcomes in many specialties.

Aneurysms could now be repaired using a stent.

Most of us were no longer wearing our nursing school caps. The white look was disappearing.

Patients had intravenous catheters that were stainless steel and gauge 16, and they stayed in for weeks. Every IV had an arm board so you couldn't possibly remove it. There were no IV pumps. I still remember the "IV Tubing Drop Factor Chart" to calculate how many drops the tubing delivered. I was always so afraid I would calculate it incorrectly. The electronic infusion device definitely provides safer, more accurate fluid administration.

There were many changes in respiratory therapy, including: IPPB, Incentive Spirometry to Nebulizers and PPV, both invasive and noninvasive. The Respiratory Therapist became so important in the management of these changes, alongside Medicine and Nursing; we recall the PR-Bennett-Bird and beyond.

When graduating from Nursing School, our class reflected on the fact that we had several men graduating with us. It seemed like such an important moment in time, to me. One of our classmates noted that he found a quote: "The world's first nursing school founded in India about 250 B.C. Only men were considered 'pure' enough to become nurses."

Around 1984, I remember hearing about Patricia Benner and her model of nursing, which was based on qualitative research. I now acknowledge her work to be so influential in nursing, providing a framework for practice as she did. Most are now aware of her study, *From Novice to Expert: Excellence and Power in Clinical Nursing Practice.*

I recall how we medically treated some diagnoses. With upper abdominal pain, a diagnosis of "duodenal ulcer," we treated them with a Levine tube inserted and a cocktail of antacids, milk and cream inserted every hour. They didn't seem to recover but after about a week of this, they went home.

1990s

We thought about our nursing colleagues in
Florida, Louisiana, and the Bahamas
as they cared for victims of category 5 Hurricane Andrew.

We remember...

The introduction of PPIs as the treatment for peptic ulcer disease. Evidence Based Practice concepts being introduced to nursing.

The Intra-Aortic Balloon Pump was about 5 feet wide and 4 feet tall and could be heard from the outside of ICU. You knew before entering the ICU that there was a patient receiving this therapy. Now it is a console that is compact, runs on Autopilot, and is most definitely more efficient when transporting someone who is that critically ill.

Nursing ratios were different. The RN's role remains the same, we use the nursing process, but I think we are more sophisticated our role.

2000s

We thought about our nursing colleagues in New York, Pennsylvania, and Washington as they cared for the victims of the worst terrorist attack in U.S. history on September 11, 2001.

We remember...

So clearly, we can all conjure what we were doing on December 31, 1999 at 11: 59 p.m. So many staff in the ICU, anxiously waiting, with extension cords in one hand and a BVM in the other. And the relief as Y2K slipped in without a hitch.

HIT came to nursing documentation.

CMS and the Joint Commission work together to bring Core Measure concepts to nursing practice.

The American Association of Colleges of Nursing recommended that all advanced practice nurses earn a Doctor of Nursing Practice degree.

SCIP measures were introduced.

The Institute for the Future of Nursing released recommendations for improved healthcare and discussion of our scope of practice.

The Nursing as Caring theory was adopted to guide our practices and the Affordable Care Act passing legislation.

The AHA supported cooling following resuscitation from cardiac arrest. Nursing played a significant role in this cohort of very sick patients. What is embedded in my memory, however, it how the patients' families responded to our aggressive care to support their loved ones.

So many predictions that nursing would be the most in-demand job.

LASER surgery reduced the need for patients to have a major surgery to remove an obstructing ureteral kidney stone. It became a 15-minute non-invasive lithotripsy.

Cesarean section deliveries could now return home in 2 days or less.

Technical changes had a positive effect on patient outcomes. The recovery phase diminished from weeks to days. The advancement of outpatient procedures decreased the need for extended hospital admissions.

Some changes occurred that would only be visible to those who worked in the OR. Major bleeding that was once controlled by clamping and tying could now be easily controlled by electro-surgical current or clips.

Respirators evolved from negative pressure Iron Lungs to the Bennet and MA ventilators. The bellows would get stuck. They worked so poorly when there was too much condensation, too, which was frequently.

The benefits of electronic medical records (EMR) for the patient and the system became more evident. They facilitate workflow, organize data and have the benefit of data mining, just to name a few.

The Gallup surveys stated, once again, that nursing consistently rated as one of the most ethical and honest professions. While it is satisfying for the public to view us as having these attributes, it's also important for us to recognize them in each other.

Epilogue

Donna Horrocks

Within the discipline of nursing, two important categories for knowledge are the empirical and the esthetic. These concern the science and art of nursing, respectively. Nursing theorists also stress the importance of personal and ethical knowledge. In becoming nurses, emerging professionals learn to identify these ways of knowing. From the newest novice to the best trained expert, there are patterns in nurses' forms of knowledge. Categorizing these ways of knowing might help in theorizing elements of practice. Yet nursing is not merely a job nor is it a philosophical project. Arguably, the lived experience of how these forms of knowledge create a unique type of professional synergy is less well theorized.

In telling our stories to one another, we have at the very least come to a deeper understanding of the esthetic, since our concern was not so much to dwell on empirical practice. Perhaps it's the uniqueness of what we do that allows us to describe and feel our experiences in this way. For my part, coming to a deeper understanding of my colleagues' journeys in the profession was a true labor of love. During this process, I could often be found anxiously perched over my inbox, just waiting for emails to arrive from my colleagues. When a new one would come in, I was thrilled.

As these stories moved from separate emails, notes, and Word documents into the shape of a book, I became further convinced that each and every one needed to be told and shared. I also quickly saw that this is not a collective biography. Nor is it strictly a reflection on a profession. This project is more like a mosaic. We could take each tile apart and inspect it, but it would not tell us very much about the project or our field of work overall. Taking a step back, and letting the light pass through, we see so much more than a string of unforgettable moments and lessons learned.

The approach of these stories, at times, seemed descriptive or autobiographical. Yet as they came together, the end result, the whole that they formed, is interpretive. These stories are often layered, because in nursing, writing about even your most intimate, personal experience still involves others. This project allowed us to come to a new understanding, together, of what being a nurse has meant to us. All of those pieces melded into something truly valuable to the world of nursing.

Notably, while nurses are trained to write and extensively document their practice, not everyone who is featured in this book wanted to write his or her own story. Some were collected orally instead. One such story began with a promise: "I'll write the story if you tell it." At the time, we were sitting, chatting, and eating as colleagues, just as we have for many years. But this was different from many of our earlier meals. We were not sitting with half-warmed holiday food or cafeteria trays. The beckoning call of beeping machines and crises were not mere minutes away; we had all the time in the world. We were enjoying a good meal and wine.

Away from the chaos of intensive care, my peers wanted to talk and I wanted to listen. I never saw this as something I would do alone. The perspective of my peers is critical; they look at the veins, they know. So, pen in hand, they talk, I scribble. I find myself listening more than scribbling, though. I'm looking, too, but not at the veins, not now. I watch with pride. These people in my life are irreplaceable, I think to myself. It is not just them—it is all of my colleagues, the ones from critical care, the ones from education, the ones that have cared for me—they bring out the best in me, and I think, in each other.

We constantly talk about how difficult our role of nursing is, but we look at each other as though it was easy and most often, we admit we could not have chosen a better life. Then we argue. There are subtle disagreements about what room a particular patient was in and who really had the hardest assignment. But then we all agree wholeheartedly about how much someone suffered, how we did our best, and how much we hoped someone would survive that horrible accident or that devastating infection. It is this dichotomy that interests me. We care about parsing the details, yet we also have much bigger concerns. As we look back, we are not dissecting these cases academically. No, it is a profound emotional pull to them that brings us back to visceral moments.

During the meal, one colleague turned to me with tears in her eyes. "I'll never forget what you said to him, over and over," she recalls. "I was in the next room and I could hear you. You kept telling him he was safe, he was out of the fire, he was in the hospital, and that you cared about him." As I looked at her, bringing myself back to that same moment, I remember thinking that sometimes our tears come so easily. Sometimes it takes a lot. You never know as a nurse. During this dinner, I know exactly who she is talking about, even though it was so many years ago. I remember this patient, just like all of the others. I remember him because I admired how brave he must have been to find his way out of that burning building. It was practically intuitive to give him pain relief, monitor his vital signs, and look for shock and early infection. This is clinical practice; all of these steps might mean the difference between life and death.

Yet nurses also need to attend to life in other ways—I somehow knew it was vital that I say the right things to him, and that this may be just as important to his survival. He needed to know he was out of the fire and safe. I tell her all of this and more. We argue over which room he was in. I know he was somewhere different than where she has recalled because she kept coming through the middle of the unit to help me. I needed her more than ever that day. There have been other times we have needed each other. She never failed to help me when a severe fracture left me in bed and then in a wheelchair for months.

Our talk circles around these personal times and the sickest patients we have seen, as well as their recoveries. We remember the patient who was so critical he eventually had a heart transplant, how he scared us when he would test the battery in his VAD that was attached to his aorta. We talked about caring for our neighbors, our friends, and our loved ones. We mentioned our responsibility to not only their health, but the responsibility to protect them, in confidence. Even now, in that restaurant, we change names, and we sit alone.

I came hoping for a great story and many unfold without effort. I silently sum it all up, as my colleagues sum up the bill. Perhaps we can chalk it up to EQ, the capacity for emotional intelligence, I am thinking. Finally, I thought we might be done for the evening. All of the meals were cleared away and my notebook tucked in my bag. Even though I wrote very little, I have gotten some great stories, and I am grateful. On the way out one of my colleagues says "it's all about the johnnie, you know. There's a lot to be said about it. No matter if you call it a johnnie or a gown, you are equalized. You're not related, you're not rich, and you're not poor." We all nod in agreement. Then someone else blurts out: "You just care about them the same way you would your own grandmother. It's simple." We all agree again.

Full of heavy meals and wine, it was probably not the best time to become philosophical, but I had to ask them how nursing impacted their lives. They indulged me, thankfully. One colleague says she thinks it has made her realize how short life can be. One states she doesn't just think, no, she knows that her friendships in nursing are the core to her life. I am listening, but still thinking about the patient who was burned. "I didn't have to think about it," I tell them. "It was reflection, the process that allows us to look at experiences from the past to impact our next decision."

Years before, I had cared for burn victims and could still remember them being so fearful they were still on fire. A very wise nurse told me then, "be sure to keep explaining to your patient that he is safe, that he will have pain, but he is no longer burning, he is out of the fire." Reflection has always been important in nursing; it supports critical thinking. It allows us to use our nursing process to benefit the one reason we really have our careers: the patients. As I say goodnight to my colleagues, these incredible nurses, I am also convinced that reflection is important for collegiality.

The stories they and others have shared for this book have both historical and personal dimensions. They show how the role of a nurse has changed. In ways big and small, nurses do not occupy the same professional space as they once did. Still, these stories show that nurses have always known the importance of evidence, even when we called it something different. As we advanced in our education, studying the science of nursing and theoretical frameworks, and as we obtained advanced degrees and certifications, we did earn respect for their importance in quality care. While the historical reflections have shown immense changes in nursing practice, the personal reflections do not chart similarly dramatic changes. Nurses with less than one year of being a professional feel the same as those with more than 50 years.

As I read the stories sent to me, and as I sat with some of the authors in this book, I saw that through personal reflection, we have always known what it means to be a nurse. On some level, we have long shared a sense of one another's importance and the value of advocacy. Over time, what's different is that nurses have gained the skills required to climb professional ladders. Out of more than forty authors in this book, there are dozens of various types of nursing certifications, many advanced degrees, quality certifications, Six Sigma distinctions, and other important benchmarks. Some have become leaders in specific realms, earning distinction in leadership, gerontology, critical care, emergency nursing, advanced practice and many more. All have worked to show a commitment to the responsibilities that go beyond the patient...... to our colleagues and the profession itself.

Nurses are right to be proud of the letters preceding or following their names. But they also ought to be proud of the informal titles they earn in providing care to each other. One has to really earn the title of leader in relation to other nurses. This means giving back, both to the institutions we work within and the communities they serve. It also means caring for each other's family members and one another in times of serious illness. I know that symbols of our care appear on plaques in shiny hallways and bricks laid on worn walkways. Our names and credentials are proudly displayed on not only institutional policies, but state-wide policies. Proof of our practice also walks among us, in families reunited after illness and in the form of babies named after a caregiver, babies who would now be grown themselves.

In collecting these stories, I am reminded of these many accomplishments. But the true evidence is not in any pin, framed certificate, or degree. In watching, listening to, and writing with my colleagues, I have learned that we are a proud group, but we are also humble. This work teaches you to be humbled by the courage and strength in other human beings. We have not been motivated to write this book by a boastful pride. No, we write and share because we have a deep sense of dignity and a drive to show that we are just a small representation of our profession. Perhaps that, as much as anything, is the spirit of nursing.

Contributors

Kristine Batty is a Nurse Practitioner. Her practice specializes in Diabetes Care.

Kelly Baxter is a Family Nurse Practitioner practicing in Palliative Care at a community hospital. She has been a nurse for more than 10 years.

Denise Bezila has a 35-year career in critical care, cardiology, and education. She is currently a Quality Specialist working to improve healthcare for veterans.

Patricia Bonzagni has been in critical care most of her career. Currently she is working in Management in Diagnostic Cardiology. She has been a nurse for more than 38 years.

Jeannine Borozny recently retired, but spent her entire 49-year career in the Operating Room arena functioning in many different capacities such as staff, management and a First Assist.

Rebecca Carley is a Nurse Practitioner caring for underserved populations. In addition, she is an Associate Clinical Professor in a graduate program. She has been a nurse for more than 38 years.

Linda Del Vecchio-Gilbert is a Nurse Practitioner who cares for children and is also faculty in undergraduate education.

Robert Desrosiers is a Family Nurse Practitioner who is an Assistant Chief Nurse in a nursing program. He has been a nurse for more than 8 years.

Pam DiMascio has worked in nursing education. She is now a Quality Improvement Specialist in a non-profit community healthcare facility. She has been in the career of nursing for 35 years.

Donna Dupuis is a Director of Nursing at a community healthcare center. She has been a nurse for more than 40 years.

Lucille Ferrer is recently retired from nursing. Her career took her from the Operating Room to geriatric long-term care. She has more than 15 years of experience as a nurse.

Leiah Gallagher is a new graduate nurse, working as a staff RN on a Medical-Surgical unit.

Marla Goulart has been in management, but recently has taken a role as an Infection Preventionist. She has been a nurse 13 years.

Allison Horrocks is a historian who served as the editor for this project. She is the proud daughter of a nurse.

Donna Horrocks has 45 years of nursing practice. She is a Clinical Nurse Specialist and works as a professor at both the undergraduate and graduate level of nursing, as well as teaching critical care.

Lisa Johnson's 40 years in nursing has taken her from geriatrics, cardiac care, and critical care, to more recently, a role in preadmission testing.

Rachel Jones works in an acute care hospital emergency department. She has been an RN for 5 years.

Rebecca Jones is currently working in Care Management; she has been in management and staff nursing for a total of 23 years as a nurse.

Elaine Joyal has had a career of appreciation for quality nursing. This has brought her from Administrative roles to Magnet designation Consultant. She has been a nurse for 37 years.

Linda Lambert's 40-year career has been in Infusion Therapy, nursing administration, and most recently, Nursing Academic Fieldwork, where she serves as a Coordinator.

Kristina Lambert is a Family Nurse Practitioner who is a provider in Women's Care and also Faculty in undergraduate nursing. She has been a nurse 14 years.

Mary Lavin is a Family Nurse Practitioner who is an Associate clinical Professor in nursing graduate studies, with more than 40 years' experience as a nurse.

Shelley MacDonald has been a nurse more than 40 years. Her most recent role was as a Chief Nursing Officer.

Michelle Mallon has more than 38 years specializing in nursing, from Surgical Care, to Administration, to currently, education.

Alisha Mal has been an emergency room nurse, and has been in management in both inpatient and emergency departments, dialysis. She has been a nurse 25 years.

Colleen Moynihan has been an RN for more than 45 years; her career stretches from intermediate care, cardiac care inpatient.

Deborah Myers has worked in critical care, cardiac care, and most recently research. She has been a nurse 22 years.

Rebekah Jean Myers is an Associate Technical Animator in video. She served as the illustrator for this book and the Spirit of Nursing project.

Ellen O'Rourke has worked in Pediatrics, home care for disabled children and adult step-down level of care. She has been a nurse 37 years.

Anabela O'Shea is an emergency room RN in a community hospital, having more than 15 years in nursing practice.

Darlene Noret is an Advanced Practice nurse who is a a Director of Nursing at the university level.

Kathleen O'Connell has worked in Oncology and currently is a Director of Infection Prevention.

Angela Quarters is a Clinical Coordinator on a surgical unit. She was previously in Quality, education and PI, for a total of 26 years.

Deborah Quirk is in a fairly new role as an Infection Preventionist, after 34 years at the bedside, including critical care and oncology.

Elizabeth Raposa teaches both graduate and undergraduate levels of nursing, and she is a critical care Nurse Practitioner. She has been a nurse for 13 years.

Barbara Saleeba recently retired from Rehabilitative / Restorative nursing after 45 years.

Linda Tierney is recently retired from nursing after 44 years. She was working in college health and education. She volunteers with R.I. Fire Chiefs Honor Flight.

Karen Treloar spent most of her 48 year career in critical care; she is currently a wound care specialist in skilled care.

Cynthia Votto is an RN in two arenas, one being inpatient Utilization Review and the other, clinical education at the undergraduate level.

Rosemary Walker worked as a nurse in various settings, including Medical-Surgical and cardiac nursing for more than 40 years.

Virginia Wilcox enjoys the challenges of a Director role in Critical Care and Hemodialysis. She has more than 45 years as an RN.

Dianna Wantoch works in Risk Management, but in the past has been active in Patient Safety and Performance Improvement. She has been a nurse for more than 30 years.

Karen Zarlenga has been a nurse for more than 35 years; her background includes cardiac and diabetes disease management. She is working as an educator for diabetes management.

Suggested Reading

Bartholomew, K. (2006). *Ending Nurse to Nurse Hostility.* Marblehead: HCPro.

Benner, P. (2001). *From Novice to Expert: Excellence and Power in Clinical Nursing Practice.* New Jersey: Prentice Hall.

Kim, S. (2000). *The Nature of Theoretical Thinking in Nursing.* New York: Springer.

Donahue, P. (2010) *Nursing, the Finest Art.* St. Louis: Mosby.

Newhouse, R., Dearholt, S., Poe, S., Pugh, L., White, K. (2007). *Johns Hopkins Nursing Evidence Based Practice Model and Guidelines.* Indianapolis: Sigma Theta Tau International.

Nightingale, F. (1918). *Notes on Nursing. What it is, What it is not.* New York: Barnes and Noble Books.

Wells, H. (1955). *Cherry Ames, Boarding School Nurse.* New York: Grosset & Dunlap.

Woodham-Smith, C. (1951). *Florence Nightingale. London*: Whitefriars Press.